—LIVING WITH—
CHRONIC
FATIGUE
SYNDROME

LIVING WITH

CHRONIC FATIGUE SYNDROME

A Personal Story
of the Struggle for Recovery

TIMOTHY KENNY

THUNDER'S MOUTH PRESS

First edition
First printing, 1994

Published by
Thunder's Mouth Press
632 Broadway, 7th Floor
New York, NY 10012

Excerpt from "Unraveling Mystery of 'Yuppie Flu.'"
Copyright 1990 USA Today. Reprinted with permission.

Lines from "Trying to Reason with Hurricane Season" by Jimmy Buffett.
Copyright MCA Music Publishing. Used by permission.

Lines from "Dust in the Wind" by Kerry Livgren.
Copyright 1980 EMI Publishing. Used by permission.

LIBRARY OF CONGRESS CATALOGING-IN-PUBLICATION DATA
Kenny, Timothy P.
   Living with chronic fatigue syndrome: a personal story of the struggle for recovery
   / Timothy Kenny.—1st ed.
      p.   cm.
   Includes bibliographical references and index.
   ISBN 1-56025-075-5 : $12.95
   1. Kenny, Timothy—Health.   2. Chronic fatigue syndrome—Patients—United
   States—Biography.   I. Title
RB150.F37K46   1994
616'.047—dc20   93-46715
[B]   CIP

Printed in the United States of America

Distributed by
Publishers Group West
4065 Hollis Street
Emeryville, CA 94608
(800) 788-3123

For Hettie
who has never wavered
from her promise,
"For better or worse,
in sickness and in health."

Oh, that I were as in months gone by . . .
As I was in the prime of my days . . .
—Job, Chapter 29

ACKNOWLEDGMENTS

The idea of writing a true story of a broadcaster combatting a serious illness was actually born a year or two before I became sick. I was talking with George Anderson, a friend and tremendous supporter of my career. George was then president of Diversified Communications' broadcasting division, making him my boss's boss. He was ill with multiple sclerosis.

I was doing a poor job of trying to think of what to say to George about still having a constructive life, when I muttered, "If something like that ever happened to me, I suppose I'd end up writing about it. Maybe that would be a way to encourage other people."

Well, something like that did happen to me, and I did end up writing about it. Thanks, George, and continued best wishes in your own struggle.

Another friend at Diversified, Liz Crosby, actually got me thinking about translating my thoughts into words in the weeks after my forced departure from the company. Liz lent me a couple of essays that really moved me, and I began to wonder if I could come up with similar verbal snapshots to share with others.

When it came to overall everyday support on this project and just making it through five years of illness, my wife Hettie tops the list. Hettie has never wavered, she's never doubted that these years I thought were wasted would account for something valuable and positive, and she's never failed to inspire me. Hundreds of nights, she has fallen asleep alone to the sound of my clicking keyboard, but she has never complained. When I first read the essays that Liz sent me, it was Hettie who urged me to consider writing myself.

My literary agent and friend, Jim Cypher, deserves thanks for sticking with me and the vision of my project for nearly two years—about twenty-three months longer than anyone else would have. In fact, Jim helped me translate my original notion of this book from random thoughts and writings into something sensible.

My brother Bob has been a real supporter, too. His daily phone calls in the weeks and months after leaving my job always came at a time when I felt the world slipping away, and I'm convinced today that his thread of communication was more important then either of us knew at the time.

Via long distance, the world's greatest TV meteorologist and my most loyal friend, Tommy Sorrells, made the phone company very rich as he stood by me, never for a moment doubting two very important outcomes: First, that I would get well someday, and, second, that I would see this book published. So far, he's batting .500 on those predictions, but Tommy's excellent forecasting instincts lead me to believe there's plenty of sunshine still to come in my future.

Another TV friend, Clay Williams, made the time to visit me almost daily in the first painful months after we stopped working together, and his taking the time to check in on his former boss meant a great deal to me.

John Hunter, Patsy Church, and Nancy Hewitt supported me constantly with their prayers and best wishes.

Bill Oder and Ray Goff deserve thanks for their technical help and support.

The staff of The Cheney Clinic in Charlotte, North Carolina, took excellent care of me during the time I worked on this book, and they always managed to keep me smiling, no matter how crummy I felt. Thanks to you all.

Marc Iverson and the CFIDS Association of America, also in Charlotte, together with their dedicated researchers across the country, helped provide one of the most important ingredients in this project—hope.

Dr. Wayne Robertson of Charlotte was generous enough to teach me the ins and outs of computer communication. Without his help, I never would have met my agent, Jim Cypher, nor have exchanged electronic mail with many other CFS patients.

The Butler (PA), Athens (GA), and Orlando (FL) CFS support groups kindly welcomed me into their meetings to tell my story before I wrote it here, and I am grateful for the new friends I made in these wonderful organizations.

And speaking of friends, I'd like to thank the handful of you all around the country who have stayed in touch with me and continued to share your lives with me, despite the fact that I've had little to offer in return. You know who you are, and I am always thrilled to hear from you.

Thanks to my longtime employers, WPDE television and Diversified Communications, for standing by me even long after I was able to help whip up on the competition with each new rating book. Thanks, too, to my new employers, WTDR/WEZC radio and Trumper Communications, for taking a chance on a guy with half a brain. And thanks to Larry Sprinkle, WCNC-TV, and Journal Broadcasting for the chance to try a TV comeback.

Thanks to my parents and the rest of the family for their support through this difficult time. I will always be indebted to my grandfather, Daniel L. Wineland, for the letters of encouragement and instruction he wrote to me before his death.

Finally, I would like to express my gratitude to the people at Thunder's Mouth Press for agreeing that this is a story worth telling, and to editor Robert Weisser for helping bring the final version of this tale together.

CONTENTS

FOREWORD

Chronic fatigue syndrome (CFS) is an emerging and therefore controversial disorder. Although this disease was hastily labeled the "yuppie flu" in the 1980s, it respects neither person nor position. CFS does seem to strike more women than men, and perhaps more whites than blacks, but this disease crosses all socioeconomic barriers and is by no means limited to that population group called "yuppies." Sadly, many of those most profoundly affected by CFS are children.

There is a great deal we know about this disease, much that we suspect about it, and much more that is yet to be discovered.

What we know is that in virtually every patient who meets the diagnostic criteria for CFS we see evidence of a revved up or "up-regulated" immune system. Furthermore, there is up-regulation of primary antiviral immune pathways, strongly suggesting that these patients are fighting an unknown virus. In respect to immune up-regulation, one could oversimplify and describe CFS as the opposite of AIDS—we know that the HIV virus eventually shuts down the victim's immune system. In another respect, however, CFS is actually very similar to the profound immunologic up-regulation seen in early HIV infection well before the development of full-blown AIDS.

We also know that CFS causes severe problems with brain function, clouds thinking, and often strips patients of much of their intellectual capacity, all apparently because of functional brain injury.

We suspect that a novel virus may be at work in CFS, cleverly hiding from the body's immune system, which kicks into overdrive trying to defeat it. The single-agent theory is presently being pursued by only a handful of determined researchers across the country and around the world, funded almost solely by private means.

1

Most researchers, whether they believe in the single-agent theory or not, suspect that there may be other associated agents or co-factors in this illness, including most of the herpes group viruses. Heredity and environment almost certainly play a role, but here again we are running ahead of what science can prove.

CFS is controversial for many reasons, not the least of which is the search for its elusive cause or causes. The disease has also forced itself into the spotlight at a time when the government and its health organizations are grappling with the AIDS epidemic and can little afford the public notion of another mysterious epidemic. CFS has come to the attention of the medical establishment through nontraditional means—generally persistent and persuasive patients and their doctors. And the mystery of this illness has attracted the mainstream media to a debate that would otherwise be taking place among members of the medical establishment in a closed and rigid system.

Since the cause of CFS is unknown, there remains no simple test to prove its existence and no accepted treatment protocol. Hiding in the shadow of AIDS and saddled with a name that describes it poorly, CFS does not receive anywhere near the attention and research funding its seriousness demands. Caught in the middle are perhaps millions of patients who cling to every bit of news that they can get their hands on, and who fight daily against prejudice and misunderstanding for the respect and help they need.

Although I and others have been studying this disease since the mid-1980s, we still face many more questions than answers. What is the cause or causes of CFS? What treatments are most effective? Is it contagious? Is it a new disease or an old one? Is it related to AIDS in any way? Why do some people seem to recover while others only get worse? Why is there so much hostility in the government, the medical profession, and the insurance industry toward what is a very real disorder?

No doubt answers to these questions will be years in coming. At the moment, private research into CFS—as well as a painfully slow government effort—is beginning to attract some of the most talented and dedicated researchers in medicine. But at the same time, CFS is often dismissed as nonexistent by many in the medical profession.

Compassion and understanding seem to be among the elements missing from the ultimate equation that will someday be needed to solve the mystery of CFS. Indeed, much of the misunderstanding can be attributed to that name. At any given time, twenty percent of the American population claims to be fatigued, and no wonder. We live in a society in which we are constantly pushed to strive, to work hard and succeed. One of the most popular expressions of our time is "no pain, no gain." Unfortunately, there is a vast difference between common fatigue and the illness presently called chronic fatigue syndrome. Normal fatigue is treated quite simply by getting more rest. CFS is a much more complex disorder, with fatigue being only one of its many symptoms.

Naming this disease "chronic fatigue syndrome" is perhaps as great an error as was calling AIDS "gay cancer" in the early days of that illness. It is just as inappropriate as calling pneumonia "chronic cough syndrome." Characterizing this illness by just one of its symptoms—fatigue—immediately blocks access to understanding and investigation, and gives patients a label that often brings open hostility from their employers, their friends and families, their insurance carriers, and even the very physicians who have known and treated them for years. After all, every one of us has been tired, and most of us have gotten over it.

Despite all of the controversy and misunderstanding, there is a single striking and convincing argument that CFS is real and must be reckoned with: the thousands of patients from around the country and their remarkably similar stories. From sufferer to sufferer, there is an incredible resonance as they talk about this destructive experience no matter where they live, no matter their levels of sophistication or education, and no matter how skeptical the listener. These patients' own words are the most compelling evidence of the existence and magnitude of chronic fatigue syndrome.

The story you are about to read by and about one such patient is not unique, though unfortunately it has not been told often enough for most people to take notice. It is a story of an energetic, ambitious person suddenly sapped of his strength, his intellect, his health, his career, and most of what else made up his very identity. In that respect, Tim Kenny's story is typical of the CFS patient experience. What is unique is that he has been able to reconstruct and retell in dramatic detail the onset and progression of his illness, and to share the feelings that accompanied the unwelcome encroachment of CFS into his life.

This book can be important to CFS patients, their families and friends, and even to the vocal skeptics who deny the reality of CFS. As I have noted, it is in meeting the CFS patient on a personal level—as you will in this book—that one becomes utterly convinced of the reality of this illness, the total devastation it can bring, and the urgent need for answers to this medical mystery.

Paul R. Cheney, M.D., Ph.D.
The Cheney Clinic
Charlotte, North Carolina

PREFACE

Why have I written a story about myself, when doing so is contrary to my experience and inclination as a journalist?

I have done this because telling my own story is the most expedient way to illustrate the experience of chronic fatigue syndrome, an experience that remains terribly misunderstood and often openly doubted and ridiculed.

I have also written my own story because, as I have told it in person to other CFS patients in support group meetings around the country, I have seen heads nod and eyes mist at the mention of shared experiences. And in these meetings—listening to the words of others more than listening to my own—I have come to learn that perhaps the simplest form of support is just knowing that someone else has been where you have been and feels what you feel.

If you are in the grips of CFS, this is very much your story, too. As they said in the old television police show, "only the names have been changed."

You may not recognize the names of the friends I have written about, but you will meet people you know in this book. You may have worked at a job much different from mine, but you will find your workplace and your co-workers in here, too. You will also be painfully reacquainted with some of the doctors you have met along this journey, and you will read about the same frustrations you may have endured from close-minded medical professionals who could have made a difference but chose not to.

In this book about me, you will find reminders of your own personal losses, your own disappointments and sadness, and the other damage and destruction that CFS may have caused in your life.

But more than all of that, I hope you will find—in this story about me—that part of yourself that has kept you fighting and will see you through this illness. That's the part of my story that I have been fortunate enough to share with CFS support groups when my health permits me to travel, and that's the part of my story that kept me awake for a year writing this book. It's the part we are all eager to share, if only we had the energy, if only we could find the words, if only we could recall the details.

As I have written this story, I have had to rely upon much more than my own elusive recollections of those details, because CFS has taken so much of my memory. As I used to do as a reporter, I interviewed those who have witnessed my decline and my illness. I have pored over hospital records, insurance documents, work calendars, and business, personal, and medical correspondence. And even though I have actually lived the nightmare of this disease, it has been only in objectively reviewing this material and writing this book that I have been able to fully grasp the absolute and total impact this disease has had on my life. I have also spent a great deal of time in one-on-one conversations with other CFS patients, and those discussions have fueled my determination to complete this project.

I am more convinced than ever—and I want to tell everyone who will listen—that we are not quitters, we are not burned out, and we are not "looking for attention." We are sick, and we want to get our lives back.

Although I guardedly use the word *recovery* in the title and in the closing chapter of this book, you will not find a spontaneous miracle cure here. I have been looking for one for years, at great pain and expense, and I have yet to find it.

The illness I describe in this book is known by several names in the United States and around the world. Most patients, informed physicians, researchers, and patient advocacy groups in the United States have adopted the name chronic fatigue and immune dysfunction syndrome (CFIDS). The U.S. government's health organizations, however, still refer to it simply as chronic fatigue syndrome (CFS). In other countries, it is called myalgic encephalomyelitis (ME).

While I believe CFIDS and ME to be more appropriate names,

in the interest of consistency, I use CFS throughout this work, hoping eagerly that a better, more appropriate name will soon be universally adopted.

Please share this book with your family and friends who have supported you, as well as with those who may have doubted you. I hope and honestly believe—in this story about me—they will all come to a better understanding of what *you* have been through.

Timothy Kenny

For more information about CFS/CFIDS/ME, contact
The CFIDS Association of America
P.O. Box 220398
Charlotte, NC 28222
800-442-3437

A portion of the proceeds from the sale of this book will fund ongoing medical research sponsored by the CFIDS Association of America.

1

DUST IN THE WIND

On Thursday, September 14, 1989, Accu-Weather sales manager Sheldon Levine was proudly showing his company's latest weather graphics computer to me. I was the newly appointed news director at television station WPDE, serving the resort area market around Myrtle Beach, South Carolina. I was in Kansas City for an annual convention of news executives, and booths of companies like Levine's packed the convention center. I was looking for something like the Accu-Weather computer to help improve our weather presentation. I was our station's backup weathercaster, and I was also a pilot. As a part-time television personality, my credibility depended on getting the weather right. As a pilot, my life depended on it.

"Can you show me a satellite picture?" I asked Levine.

"No problem," he answered confidently. "Let's take a look at the mid-Atlantic. There's something interesting going on out there."

He punched a few buttons and the color screen began to fill with the blue-and-white images of the Atlantic Ocean, partially covered by a distinct cloud pattern.

"Wow! What's that?" I asked, pointing to the counterclockwise spiral just off the African coast. I could tell that it was probably the beginnings of a hurricane.

"It's a new storm—I think they're gonna call it Hugo," Sheldon answered. He tapped expertly on the keyboard and continued talking about his new computer system.

I wasn't listening. I was a thousand miles away from my new

responsibilities as news director, and the thought of a possible hurricane made me nervous. Along the Southeast coast, hurricanes and tropical storms are a threat from May until October every year. This year, in a planning meeting with my boss, station manager Bill Christian, I had even predicted the "big one" would hit us on September 23.

Now I looked at Hugo and did some quick calculating. If the storm tracked toward South Carolina, it would hit about September 23. (As it turned out, the storm of the decade hit us head-on at midnight on Friday, September 22.) I left Levine in mid-presentation and called Bill in South Carolina.

"I think we should have a department head meeting as soon as I get back," I said. "How about Monday afternoon?"

"Whatever you think," Bill answered.

I was pleased that he took my hunch so seriously, but I was also concerned about the possibility of crying "wolf" so soon in my new position. Bill had promoted me from managing the one-person (me) promotion department to heading the station's largest and most visible department only weeks earlier. Bill had told me that he was promoting me because he trusted my instincts, my performance under pressure, and my planning. I wanted to follow my instincts, but I didn't want to jump the gun and look like a fool.

"You're not just lucky in the news business," Bill had told me, "you set yourself up to be lucky." Like me, Bill wanted to be ready for the big stories long before they actually happened. The middle of a disaster is no time to come up with a news plan.

I caught a late flight home from Kansas City on Sunday. Resisting the temptation to sleep in Monday morning, I rushed in to work. I cornered Bill even before he had finished reading the morning newspaper.

"This really could be the big one," I said. I showed Bill the latest storm coordinates, explained to him the upper atmosphere steering currents and the computer models for landfall, and we quickly arrived at the consensus that precautions were definitely in order; my concern was now *our* concern.

We both knew the potential fallout from overreacting to a hurricane so far away. We could hurt the station's (and Bill's and my) reputation and credibility if we went on the air and alarmed people about Hugo unnecessarily. Still, Bill and I agreed to set ourselves up to be lucky just in case the storm might hit us.

We decided not to summon all of the station's department heads together with the storm's landfall still so uncertain. Instead we called a meeting of what I called the PEONs: the heads of Promotion, Engineering, Operations, and News. Bill called it the OPEN group, but I had jokingly renamed us PEON, and that name stuck.

After a few opening remarks, Bill turned the meeting over to me. "Hugo is a big storm, expected to get even bigger," I began. No one really reacted; they hadn't even heard of Hugo until that meeting. Besides, they'd all heard this before. We had already had a false alarm earlier in the summer when another hurricane shadow-boxed our coastline before moving harmlessly into the North Atlantic. I sensed that no one but Bill and I were taking this meeting—and Hugo—very seriously. It is the same problem that law enforcement authorities face when they try to evacuate a coastal community: "The last storm didn't get us, so why should this one?"

"We need to be ready," I continued, looking in Bill's direction for support. "I just have a feeling that Hugo could be coming our way." I conceded that the computer models still showed the storm had just as great a chance of hitting Florida or even turning away from the mainland altogether. But I continued making my case, turning to Bill Elks, our chief engineer.

"Bill, let's order a generator for the Myrtle Beach studio and stockpile some fuel. We already have generators here at the main studio and at the transmitter, right?"

He nodded, taking notes and glancing to Bill for the silent nod that turned my suggestions into orders.

"Okay, let's make sure we have plenty of fuel for all of the generators," I continued. I'd reported from one hurricane a few years earlier, and I knew that power outages were common enough to foil even the best-laid plans. (To stay on the air during Hurricane Diana in 1985, I'd "acquired" aviation gasoline for my thirsty news car and portable transmitter. All of the conventional gas stations were useless after the electricity went off.)

"What about the live trucks?" I asked, probing the status of our two mobile units that could go on the air from anywhere in our coverage area. "How much wind can the antennas take?"

"Twenty, maybe twenty-five miles an hour, not much more," Elks answered. Each truck had a mast that telescoped sixty feet into the air when fully extended, supporting a dish-shaped microwave antenna.

"That won't do," I said. "We have to show this storm *live* if people are going to take it seriously. What about designing some portable guy wires . . . maybe some ropes?"

Elks nodded, jotting more notes. "I don't know if it's been done before, but if there's somewhere to anchor them, it could work."

"And the fixed microwave tower at the beach," I continued, "how much wind can that take?"

"Maybe eighty or a hundred miles an hour," he answered. Bill was nearly thirty years older than I, a lifelong coastal resident, and a veteran of many hurricanes. Hurricane winds could easily top that speed, but the tower, used to relay signals from our coastal Myrtle Beach studio to our main facility inland, could not be strengthened without major engineering effort, and there wouldn't be time.

"And the main tower?" I asked.

This multimillion-dollar, two-thousand-foot engineering marvel was our station's lifeblood. Without it, we weren't a TV station anymore—we couldn't transmit a thirty-second ad. "It'll hold," Elks said, and I took his word for it.

"Promotion," I continued down my checklist. "We need to get promos on the air telling people we're the *official* Hugo station, that WPDE will have all the up-to-the-minute information and live reports throughout the storm."

"Can we actually say we're the 'official' hurricane station?" someone asked.

"We *should* say it," I answered, "before the competition thinks of it."

Someone else suggested installing a special hurricane tracking telephone line with a recording of the latest storm coordinates. This would help ease the burden on our main switchboard. Thus, our hurricane hotline was born. Our meteorologist would update the recording every few hours.

Operations was next. "Can we get round-the-clock crews in about two days?" I asked Carl Jackson. "If Hugo is a threat, we'll know by then. Directors, graphics, camera people, the works?" Carl silently made some notes, and I assumed that meant reluctant agreement.

"OK . . . so what about news?" Bill Christian asked, turning the spotlight on me. No one had heard me mention my own plans. All the support in the world from the other departments was of no use if news couldn't keep functioning under the rigors of a major storm. Bill had taken a chance by moving a thirty-year-old into the position of news director. Our station had developed a bad reputation of dropping the ball on the Big Story, and Bill wasn't about to allow me the opportunity to continue that miserable tradition.

"We'll be ready," I answered. "I've had a hurricane plan drawn up since May, and I updated it this morning. I'll have a memo out to the entire staff with specific assignments by the end of the day." Having spent twenty hours reporting from Diana in 1985, I thought I knew what a hurricane was: lots of windy rain that finally moves on leaving everyone feeling lucky. Looking back on that PEON meeting, I realize that I had no idea what we would endure a week later. Hugo nearly cost some of us our lives, and certainly changed us all forever. As the meeting drew to a close, I could not have imagined the horror that awaited us all. "Hope for the best, plan for the worst," I stressed—one of my favorite operational clichés.

I wanted to end on something of an upbeat note, since I could tell that everyone thought I was already taking this whole Hugo thing too seriously.

"Dry socks," I said, closing my notepad. "Dry socks are the key to covering any hurricane. Trust me, I've been through this before. Everybody bring extra socks, and we'll be fine."

"Dry socks" would be repeated many times for mild comic

relief in the coming hours as Hugo continued its ominous track toward us.

The rest of the PEON group smiled at my remark, no doubt thinking that Hugo would miss us as the rest of the major storms had recently. But the uneasy feeling I'd first experienced in Kansas City remained with me as the hours passed.

I didn't sleep well that night. I hadn't been sleeping well for nearly a year, but that night, at least, I had a good reason.

By the next Wednesday, September 20, Hugo had done nothing to lessen my apprehension. The storm continued to strengthen, stalking steadily toward the South Carolina coast. I had officially enacted my Hurricane Operation Plan that morning, and I'd relocated from our main building in Florence, seventy miles inland, to our Myrtle Beach studio, two miles from the coast, where about a quarter of our sixty-person staff would join me. From here, I'd lead our coverage in the field. Bill Christian and my executive producer, Tom Knight, would lead the remainder of the staff in Florence. As events progressed, Bill and Tom played larger and larger roles. Going in, we expected to make several hourly reports about the wind and rain along the coast, with little or no real disruption of our usual broadcasting schedule. The way the week unfolded, though, virtually all of our programming was produced on the fly, and I spent much of my time in the midst of the fury of the storm and the aftermath, in no position to make all of the minute-by-minute decisions. Thanks to Bill and Tom, "hope for the best, plan for the worst" worked superbly.

Tuesday night, too, had been sleepless, as I tossed and turned, contemplating a face-to-face with Hugo. I had packed several days' clothes (including plenty of socks), and had briefed the staff on their assignments before I headed for the beach. By then, Hugo's landfall had been narrowed to a several-hundred-mile stretch of densely populated coastline in the Southeast. Myrtle Beach sat squarely in the center of that area. Our entire staff was now taking Hugo seriously.

The phones at both of our studios were ringing off the hook with calls from anxious viewers. Each new National Hurricane

Center projection narrowed landfall closer and closer to our region. The Center's director, Dr. Bob Sheets, was live on our news that night at six o'clock.

"Hurricane Hugo is continuing to strengthen, and its eye is becoming more well-defined," he told our audience, pointing at computer-enhanced satellite images of the storm on a television monitor. By now, Sheets was giving interviews only to the TV markets that Hugo was most likely to hit.

I stayed with one of our mobile units on the oceanfront until after the 11:00 P.M. news, acting partly as director, partly as producer, and still being consulted from our main studio on the unfolding drama. I even went on the air myself to add an experienced face to our crew of young reporters.

Wednesday was another sleepless night. Was everything in order? Safety was vital, and I had even formed an evacuation plan for our staff. I wasn't trying to be a hero, but I made it known that I'd be among the last to take refuge—at least I'd been in a hurricane before and I had studied weather. Everyone's worst nightmare was a huge storm surge that could drown anyone within several blocks of Myrtle Beach's Ocean Boulevard. I worried that if it came in the darkness, its assault might be unnoticed until it was too late.

Had I done everything I could? Was everyone in the right place? Were we completely ready? Was *I* completely ready? Did I have the strength to make it through this?

I reminded myself that I was in charge, and I *had to* have the strength. My body had been protesting nearly everything I pushed it to do lately. I couldn't fail here; this was our TV station's chance to outshine the competition and prove that we were the best. I had to make it through for a more important reason—people's lives were at stake. I felt that the lives of not only those on my staff, but also the residents of the area, were riding on my back.

On Thursday, September 21, I was on the beach at sunrise, reporting live in the eerie early morning calmness. Wispy white clouds high in the sky bore no hint of what was just eighteen hours away, but the official tracking data left little room for doubt. If Hugo didn't hit us head-on, we now knew it would still shake us up. I ordered the newly designed guy wires attached to the mobile unit's antenna mast.

The normally blue Atlantic was already churning an ominous gray, and the waves were breaking higher than on a typical morning. But I couldn't yet visualize the monster that would soon swallow up the ground upon which I now stood—it was still beyond the horizon.

We aired hourly updates throughout the morning, and by afternoon Governor Carroll Campbell—a coastal homeowner himself—ordered a complete evacuation of the immediate shore and several blocks inland. Over the protests of the local police, we held our ground with our live trucks and our video cameras. I knew our live pictures of the storm's approach might at the very least make history. At the most, they would save lives.

We calculated that if Hugo continued on its present course at its present speed, the storm would hit land well after dark, probably around midnight. It would be nearly impossible to air live pictures of the hurricane at that hour, and it would certainly be too late for anyone to react. We had to make our case for evacuating now, while there was still light, still electricity, still time.

At noon, I did a live update alongside one of my reporters. He had confessed to me about his fear of the storm, and as I stood a few feet away from the pounding surf, I allowed as how his fear was really quite rational. (One year later, a vacationer who had been in Myrtle Beach that day tracked me down and gave me a photo of me and my camera crew doing that update. Prominently displayed now in my office, the picture reminds me daily that disaster can lurk just beyond the horizon. I look at that picture and I see a Tim Kenny who thought no force of nature was too great to conquer. How arrogant. For me, Hugo was the beginning of understanding how frail and small a human being really is.)

By the time of our 6:00 P.M. news, the weather was deteriorating rapidly, and a premature dusk had enveloped the area. Most of the dozens of news crews who were fighting for beachfront position earlier in the day had abandoned downtown Myrtle Beach. Fear, prudence—whatever caused it, courage and patience were wearing thin among the news corps. In one of the remaining crews, from a television station in upstate South Carolina, a fistfight broke out between the reporter and the satellite truck operator when the latter announced they would be abandoning their position and moving inland. Our new guy wires kept us on the air, while this crew exchanged punches and then retreated.

Just moments before the six o'clock newscast, one of our reporters dropped her heavy clipboard, and I watched it blow away like a scrap of litter. Someone scrambled after it, disappearing toward the pounding surf into the pelting rain that was now coming nearly horizontally. Standing upright was almost impossible, and our reporter held onto a railing to give her live report. I wrapped an arm around a lightpole for support.

At 6:05, Tom Sorrells, the station's meteorologist and my best friend, again interviewed Dr. Sheets via satellite from the National Hurricane Center in Florida. I watched from the wind-shaken sanctuary of our mobile truck. Hugo was now only hours away, and there was no doubt anymore about where it was heading.

"You in Myrtle Beach are directly in the path of this major storm," Sheets told our audience. Even now, hearing the tape of those words makes my skin tingle.

An hour later, as the invisible sun was setting over more tranquil territory to the west, we reluctantly moved two miles inland to our studio, away from the impending storm surge. But rather than broadcasting from inside the studio, we set up a camera position in the parking lot. We were now the only local station still showing the approach of Hugo live as it happened. I joined our reporters doing updates in the screaming wind and rain outside our studio. Hugo's full fury was just off the coast, but this early taste convinced us all that we were in for a hellish night.

I began to feel real fear. What had been a hunch several months earlier, a guess just a week before, a haunting thought one sleepless night ago, was now happening all around us, and I had absolutely no control over any of it.

I discussed our personal evacuation plan and criteria one last time with my staff still on the air in Myrtle Beach. Hugo was now a category 4 hurricane, just about as big as they come. All unnecessary personnel had already evacuated our studio and taken refuge in a sheltered hotel complex, but a few of us were determined to keep going as long as we could.

From the North Carolina line down through Myrtle Beach and on into Charleston—more than half of South Carolina's coast-line—tens of thousands of people were being evacuated, buildings were being blown down, signs were being ripped from the ground, power transformers were popping on utility poles like fireworks on the Fourth of July. We felt the wind pound our studio, shaking the walls as you might shake a towel on wash day. This was the real thing, an experience that could never be imagined no matter how carefully I planned.

At 11:30, I hurriedly instructed my last photographer, Richard Perdue, to evacuate to our agreed-upon location after a tree limb nearly crushed him outside our studio during a live update. Richard had a wife and new baby at home. At 11:45, my remaining reporter and I left, the last to evacuate our facility. The roof of the studio was heaving in the howling wind. Just as I'd seen the crew from upstate battle several hours earlier along the beach, the reporter and I argued about the decision to abandon our studio. We stood there shouting at each other even though the shrieking wind made it impossible to hear anything. Fear and helplessness sometimes make us lash out at anyone who happens to be nearby, whether innocent or not.

Shortly after we left the studio, our fixed-link microwave tower crashed to the ground, smashing the rear of our building and crushing everything in its path.

The decision to leave had been as much a practical one as it had been a safety consideration. The wind was too great for our antennas to stand, the power and phone lines had been knocked out, and repairs were impossible. The only one issue left to consider was survival.

At midnight, the center of Hurricane Hugo, with winds nearing 150 miles per hour, passed over Charleston and McClellanville to the south. We in Myrtle Beach found ourselves in the storm's deadly northeast quadrant. In the coming weeks, we were overlooked by the national media—Charleston was a much more appealing story and much easier to cover—but we were not overlooked by the mass of counterclockwise flowing wind and rain I had first feared more than a week earlier while looking at a computer in Kansas City.

Hugo tore us to shreds.

By Saturday evening, September 23, Hugo had come and gone, leaving behind $5 billion in damages to our state alone, continuing on a furious path through central North Carolina and onward as far north as Pennsylvania and New York. Thankfully, loss of life was low. The early warnings from the National Hurricane Center, the evacuation orders from Governor Campbell, and superb media information like ours had all paid off.

Throughout our coverage area, neighborhoods were picking up and digging out, and power was slowly being restored. At my own home, seventy miles inland, we would not have electricity for more than a week.

As more and more people had their utilities reconnected in the hours immediately after Hugo, calls flooded the television station asking for the latest information on the storm, the clean-up efforts, the damage, where to go for help. Before Hugo's landfall, I had thought our jobs would end the morning after what I had presumed would be a relatively harmless storm.

I was wrong: covering the actual storm was just the beginning of the job.

Saturday evening, I worked with a mobile truck along Ocean Boulevard, in nearly the same place we had done our six o'clock news just two days before. The damage there was unfathomable. All clichés used to describe the destruction had been abandoned twenty-four hours earlier. Now, the pictures were left to tell the story.

At 7:00 P.M., we went on the air from that spot with yet another special report. (We had now been doing live updates for nearly four days without a break). In this update, as in others, we showed pictures of destruction, emotion, devastation, and heroism. "Hope for the best, plan for the worst" had done little to help me antici-pate the scene that surrounded us.

As we were setting up the camera and lights for this special report, five roofing nails from blown-off shingles punctured my shoes in less than half an hour. I ripped out the nails and limped about my duties, making a mental note to get a tetanus shot when this was all over. It would be two weeks before I had the time to visit an emergency room.

By this point, most of us were stretched to our limits, in some-thing of a state of shock that had been deepened by days without sleep. We had become testy and often angry with each other. I had gone so long without sleep and had become so irritable that one of my own staff members actually drugged me as I drank a warm beer "to settle me down." I dozed for a short while from the two sleep-ing pills she had put in the beer, not knowing whether to thank her or fire her when I found out later what had happened.

One of our commercial producers, Chuck Spruill, assembled a musical montage to end that seven o'clock special report. As more and more of our audience were once again able to watch televi-sion, we kept trying to find fresh ways to recap the previous two days. Chuck's music video included some of the most amazing images of Hugo and its aftermath, and it reached deep inside my aching body and touched emotions I had been ignoring. The music was "Dust in the Wind" by the rock group Kansas, and I remember some of the most poignant lyrics from Chuck's presentation:

> Don't hang on,
> Nothing lasts forever but the earth and sky.
> Dust in the wind,
> All we are is dust in the wind.

The dramatic video, and indeed Hurricane Hugo itself, had proved as much to me, and Chuck had chosen the perfect words and music to describe what we all felt. After Hugo, we knew that we were merely dust in its giant wind, and no more. It was, for many of us, a life-changing experience.

*   *   *

Later that night, I drove home to wash some clothes and to assess the damage to my own house. I had thought that driving inland would take me to less-affected areas; that the damage would end just a few miles from the coast. Again I had underestimated Hugo. It seemed as if nothing had been spared.

In the darkness, sixty miles from the ocean and nearing my town, the devastation was everywhere, at least as bad as I had seen near the beach. I had to fight back tears those final few miles on my way home. I thought I would be finally escaping the horrible destruction, and instead I was driving deeper into it. There was no getting away from the terrible ruin. It was everywhere.

Arriving at our headquarters studio, I found Bill Christian. We had been through so much together this past week, from my call in Kansas City to the forces of nature at their worst, all the while orchestrating some of the finest live disaster coverage in the history of local television. Through Hugo and the immediate aftermath, Bill and I were in constant contact, though we were far apart, each playing his respective role professionally. It was good for two battle-weary newsmen to see each other again. I had sand in my hair and clothes and in my wet shoes, and I hadn't shaved for days. Bill appeared equally disheveled, though I can say with some confidence that we were both wearing dry socks.

I reached out to shake Bill's hand. Instead, he embraced me, and our stubbled faces brushed past each other, recording another Hugo memory I'll always remember. There was nothing to say. Without shame, we both shed tears over the loss that had taken place all around us.

Nearly two years after Hugo, on August 20, 1991, my staff sat nervously around the conference room, awaiting the meeting I had called immediately after a six o'clock newscast. A few of the faces had changed since the hurricane, but most of these people had been with me since the giant storm, when we'd all learned to respect each other and depend upon one another. In a context where friendships are often no more than an on-camera act, we had managed to become a close-knit group; sort of a family, in fact.

Perhaps it was because I was just a few years older than they and was a friend as much as a boss. Or maybe it was because I rarely stayed in my office, preferring instead to work side-by-side with them whenever possible, as I'd done in Hugo.

I also believe we were close because we had shared a common event in history and we had survived it together. Most of those people are far from South Carolina today, working in other news organizations. But they still tell me that—miserable as their jobs may have been at times—the time we spent together in South Carolina remains unique and appreciated.

They'd been wondering throughout that day in 1991 why I was summoning them for this unusual meeting, shrouded in secrecy. The top guess was that economics had forced some cutbacks at the station and I was about to deliver the bad news. This was becoming commonplace in broadcasting. Another possible reason, some of them had guessed, had something to do with my health. Eighteen months earlier, I'd been diagnosed with an illness that didn't sound too bad—chronic fatigue syndrome—and they had seen my condition worsen since then. I couldn't pull all-nighters as I used to, and I'd become something of a scatterbrain, often forgetting an order I'd issued only the day before. I'd given up the fun job of backup weathercaster because it had become too much for me. Sometimes I walked and acted like an old man, full of pain and uncertainty. Frighteningly, they'd seen me stumble and lose my balance. They knew I was participating in an experimental trial for a new drug, that I was being a human guinea pig. But I had maintained a facade of toughness, and my staff of friends had no idea just how serious my situation had become.

As soon as I began the meeting, I assured them there would be no cutbacks, no layoffs, no firings. The group heaved a collective sigh of relief. There would be one person who would be leaving, however, and that person would be me. I was too sick to continue working.

Five days earlier, in a conference with my physician and my wife Hettie, we decided that my working any longer would continue to injure my brain and my body, and I might be giving up any chance I had at ever getting well again. I had good days and bad days, but the balance was tipping more and more toward the bad. If I were to ever return to the business of wrestling with hurricanes and training talented young reporters, I needed to take immediate steps to protect my deteriorating body. While saying that to my staff, I actually knew that I would never return to be with them. There are no "sabbaticals" in broadcasting. I knew in my heart that I'd never return to that place, to those people, ever again.

In that short meeting, I bid my staff an emotional goodbye, and I did what I could to promise an easy transition for them all. The next day, with very little fanfare—it takes only moments to become a has-been in broadcasting—I cleaned out my desk and drove away with an office full of memories crammed into my tiny car. The moment was even more humbling than the painful moment on Ocean Boulevard two years earlier, when I had watched Chuck Spruill's musical presentation full of destruction and emotion. As with that instant two days after Hugo, I was emotionally overwhelmed.

What had been a hunch a long time ago, and a nagging fear more recently, had turned into an awful reality from which recovery did not seem possible. The storm had come, and it had destroyed everything. The comparison with September 1989 and Hurricane Hugo haunted me.

I was again, as I had been then, dust in the wind.

2
GREAT EXPECTATIONS

By all measures, the summer of 1988—more than a full year before Hurricane Hugo and more than three years before I would be forced out of television—promised to be the best time of my life. I was my own boss at a great television station in a great market that included some of the most beautiful weather and beaches in the Southeast. I was making more money than I'd ever thought possible, and earning more professional respect than I'd ever dreamed of.

I was relatively new to the television business, having spent a year in TV earlier in the decade and then returned to it in late 1985. Despite my limited experience, much of what I touched was turning to gold. Our little TV station that could, *was*, and I was a big part of it all. I was clearly on a roll, and so was our television station, WPDE, the ABC affiliate in the Florence/Myrtle Beach market, in the northeast corner of South Carolina.

My title then was director of station promotion, which meant I was in charge of making all the commercials you see where the TV news anchors smile at each other and hold babies at parades. I also made the short announcements that promote the next episode of, say, *Home Improvement* or some other syndicated programs. In addition to having creative oversight of these promos, I also had charge of our graphics and music and anything else that had to do with the station's image. It was a big job, but I was having a ball doing it.

Along with all of that came the especially enjoyable duty of

being the liaison with the promotion divisions at the ABC network and our program syndicators. Among other things, that
meant I got to go to Hollywood for huge parties and other func-
tions where I would actually meet the TV stars that the rest of our
station's staff only heard about. And when the stars came to our
market, it was I who arranged their visit and I who was their constant escort. It was all quite a kick for a kid who'd grown up on five
acres in the country feeding chickens and weeding the vegetable
garden, dreaming of someday making his own way to Hollywood.

I also got to write special promos that the stars would record
especially for our station to air only in our market. Considering
that my first writing job was covering high school sports for a
green-sheet newspaper that paid a penny per word, it was quite a
thrill to be writing scripts that would be taped by the likes of Peter
Jennings or Bill Cosby. My earlier dreams of Hollywood were no
more exciting than the life I was now leading.

As I'd been tuning up the station's image since being named
promotion director two and a half years earlier, I was also tuning
up my own image. The new job and prestige had given me new
incentive, and I wanted to look and act like a professional in every
way. That meant a personal image overhaul.

I had been overweight since childhood, and I set about to lose
the extra pounds. As with nearly every other project I had taken
on, I succeeded, dropping nearly forty pounds in a few months and
whipping my body into the best shape of my life. I felt great. It was
such a joy to finally have a body I could be proud of and to be able
to run side-by-side at the local health club with actual athletes.

I fully agreed with the no-pain, no-gain axiom, and had no fear
of pain. I worked out just about every day at the club, running
either early in the morning, at lunchtime, or—if the day got away
from me—late at night. I was twenty-nine, and for the first time in
my life I was beginning to feel like everything was falling into
place. I was proud of who I had become.

I was an airplane pilot, too, another accomplishment I'd only
dreamed of many years before. The previous summer had marked
three major aviation milestones for me. I'd earned my instrument
rating, I'd flown a small plane to a tiny island getaway in the

Bahamas, and I'd flown in an F-16 fighter jet with the Air Force Thunderbirds.

Life had never looked more promising, though I worked incredibly hard every day to achieve the success that had made this all possible. I thrived on the hard work, long hours, and tireless brainstorming that were paving the way for my success in television. Some of the other station department heads openly resented me because I would often sneak away for long strategy sessions with Bill Christian, the new general manager. The ideas born at such sessions inevitably resulted in positive on-air improvements and high praise from upper management. At these planning sessions, Bill and I helped hatch plans for expanding our news coverage, adding additional news and weather personnel, and earning the right to be Myrtle Beach's very own television station, something no one had figured out how to do before.

Since Myrtle Beach was halfway between the Wilmington, North Carolina and Florence, South Carolina markets, it was a city without a television identity of its own. Whichever market could make the Myrtle Beach viewers and advertisers feel more at home and earn the ratings to prove it would reap millions of dollars in new advertising revenues. Bill and I recognized this huge untapped potential and made it our top priority. (Both markets laid claim to the viewer-rich Myrtle Beach area, but the ratings services still credited that huge chunk of audience to Wilmington, and by default most of the ad money went there.) Since I had been a very successful radio reporter in Myrtle Beach a few years earlier, Bill looked upon my advice and intuition with great favor.

Bill Christian had been general manager for a year, and we clicked well after the first few awkward weeks that are a part of any management transition. Making great TV became a passion for us.

Bill was a year younger than I, at the time making him the youngest station manager in the business. Our youth and our can-do attitudes were turning WPDE from a second-rate station to the pacesetter in the market and arguably the pacesetter in the state. As a professional athlete might look back at a championship season, I fondly look back at those days and think how great it was to be on a winning team that seemed unstoppable. We just kept cranking out great ideas, and they worked. Bill and I definitely were playing in the "zone," the way a quarterback and a wide receiver might team up for a season full of highlight plays. One of the real kicks for me was crossing departmental lines and dabbling in news, my old stomping grounds. My years in radio had been full of success and adventure, and I acquired a good feel for what worked. Now in television, unfamiliar news territory, I was asked to audition for the position of backup weathercaster. Though I had never been on-camera before, I jumped at the chance to be back in the spotlight. With my new confidence, my new body, a new wardrobe, and the feeling that nothing could go wrong, I loved the chance to fill in when the main weathercaster was on vacation or called in sick.

When I was still in junior high school, I had hooked two turntables together in my bedroom and practiced being a disk jockey, "airing" simulated radio broadcasts with my mother's poodle as the only listener. I studied on my own and got an FCC license, landing my first radio job just months after graduating from high school. I had gotten my real chance to deejay on my way up the career ladder in radio, and I never forgot that thrill of being on the air. And being on television was so much more exciting than radio had ever been. People actually recognized me in public!

As WPDE's number-two weathercaster, I also had to stand by when the main weathercaster was out on a remote broadcast, say from a festival or church bazaar or Christmas tree lighting. Technical details sometimes got fouled up back then as we were just getting the feel of live shots, and at such times I'd have to jump in and do the weather when the remote signal was lost. I went on the air acting as if nothing had gone wrong and giving the weather without missing a beat.

Sometimes, just to prove I could do it, I wouldn't even *look* at the weather maps when I knew I'd be standing by. If the live shot fell through because of technical problems, I'd quickly clip on a microphone, walk onto the set, and ad lib through the entire presentation without a moment's preparation. That astounded people who saw me do it, but for me it was actually easy. Radio had taught me to ad lib, flying had taught me the weather, and I had developed a daredevil attitude somewhere along the way. Living on the edge with last-minute broadcasts became a thrill and an adrenaline rush that just couldn't be beaten. I actually *hoped* that we'd have technical problems on the live remotes, so I could jump in and do my thing. After years of hiding behind a radio microphone ashamed of my appearance, this was a seductive experience.

Once when the weathercaster was on vacation, a line of severe thunderstorms moved through our area just before the eleven o'clock news. The heavy winds and downpours made weather the top story. At two minutes before airtime, the studio took a direct lightning strike that destroyed the weather graphics computer. We normally did our weather outside, but in conditions like this the weathercaster moved indoors to avoid the danger. With only seconds before the start of the newscast, everyone was scrambling to bring me inside away from the lightning, wondering how I'd fill four minutes without any weather maps or statistics on the screen. (Not only did I have a full weather segment to fill without maps and satellite pictures, I was also scheduled to do an entire minute at the beginning of the show, briefly describing the most recent developments.)

The producer planned on my having a radar image to show, but that, too, had been destroyed in the lightning hit.

"I'm staying outside," I told the director. "This is great video! Just give it to me and I'll go with it."

At exactly eleven o'clock, our anchorman apologized for the brief power interruption that had blown up our equipment and momentarily knocked the station off the air. Then he pitched to me standing in the rain, wind, and lightning to explain the latest on the storm. I had no notes, maps, or statistics, but I had a tremendous backdrop for the top story of the night. Sheets of driving rain punctuated by bone-rattling thunder and menacing lightning helped me tell that story better than any weather maps would have, and I presented the information without missing a single detail.

The time passed in what seemed like an instant, and before I knew it the cameraman (safely inside, shooting through a hole in the wall) was giving me the signal to wrap up. It was time to pitch back inside. I'd done what they were all worried couldn't be done—but for me it was an irresistible challenge and I loved every second of it. The regular weather segment just five minutes later went every bit as well. I didn't need props to tell a story back then, and I still don't.

The next morning I received memos from the news director and the general manager, both congratulating me on the miracle I'd pulled off. *What miracle?* I thought. I'd had fun, and I secretly longed for the next chance to do the "impossible."

Monday, May 30, 1988—Memorial Day—was a company holiday. For me, that meant I could go to work wearing blue jeans instead of a suit and tie. There was always work to be done, and I never took a holiday off. I could accomplish a lot when the building was nearly empty.

Early that afternoon, a friend whom I hadn't seen for about a year called. She invited me to come visit her soon in another part of the state where she was now living. It was something we'd been talking about for months.

I glanced at my schedule for the coming week. Impossible. This was the busiest time of year for our station. "No way," I had to say, and we were both disappointed.

"What about next week?" she asked.

That was out of the question, too. I would be in Los Angeles that week for network meetings and parties.

"The week after that?"

"Nope, that won't work either," I explained. Hettie and I had planned a short vacation to the Bahamas immediately after my return from California.

"Then how about today?"

I looked at my watch. Just as I longed to go on the air with no preparation, this was my way of doing things—no planning, no props, just jump on a plane and go.

"I'll make a few calls and get right back to you," I said, the adrenaline already pumping. Maybe I would take *part* of a holiday off after all!

I dialed the airline. There was a connecting flight leaving

within the hour, with a return later that night, and another early the next morning in case I missed that flight. I absolutely *had* to be at work the next day: ABC's *Good Morning America* would be airing its weather segments from Myrtle Beach the coming Friday at my invitation, and there were dozens of details still to be handled.

I called Hettie. She knew my instant-action attitude and went along with my crazy plan. I called my friend with my flight information and then raced home to pick up an overnight kit.

My friend and I had a nice visit, a light dinner, and a chance to catch up with each other's lives. Then it was off to the airport for my connecting flight home. By midnight I was slipping back into my own bed, glad I'd made the trip but glad to be home. Spur-of-the-moment had worked again. Memorial Day had turned out to be an eighteen-hour day with four airplane rides and dinner in another town—just my way of doing things.

Tuesday was crazy. The GMA people were on the phone at least once an hour as I worked to arrange details including a satellite truck and special telephone communication lines. These New York people didn't do things the way I did—they planned *everything*. They even decided to send their own director along with their location manager. The star of the broadcast would be weathercaster Spencer Christian. The occasion for which I'd invited *Good Morning America* to Myrtle Beach was the start of the annual Sun Fun Festival, our official kickoff to summer.

Although the GMA remote was demanding most of my time, it was only one of several major projects I was producing that weekend. We were doing our own news and weather live from the beach, covering a hundred-entrant parade, and showing live what we liked to call "navel to navel" coverage of the annual bikini contest. *Then* we would begin the twenty-one-hour Children's Miracle Network Telethon, all live. Since such remote telecasts were my specialty, it was all up to me to make sure the Myrtle Beach end of everything went well.

By Wednesday, the pressures of coordinating everything were mounting exponentially. But this was life in the fast lane, I was an important component in it, and I wouldn't have it any other way. I was up to the "impossible" challenge of it all.

Then, about midway through the day, an out-of-town emergency came up involving a friend. I dropped what I was doing, drove three hours to check on the situation, turned around less than a half hour later and drove back. That was an impulsive thing to do, considering everything else I had to do that week. But I never lacked for acting on impulse, and when the call came, I jumped. The afternoon and evening were gone, and I still had much work to do.

On the way home I called Hettie to check for messages.

"The GMA producer called. There are some changes they want to make. Here's her home number," Hettie relayed.

It was after ten o'clock at night and I was still more than two hours from home, but there from that phone booth I worked through the changes ABC wanted.

By 1:00 A.M. I was finally in bed, my heart still racing from the hurry-up trip and anticipation of the network people's arrival the next day.

Thursday brought more details, more problems, more particulars to be worked out, plus the normal everyday effort that came with my job. By noon I'd made all the last-minute assignments and covered every technical angle I could anticipate. I went home and packed, then drove the seventy miles to Myrtle Beach Jetport to meet Spencer Christian and his crew. I got to the gate about two minutes before the plane landed, but as a good host I acted as if there were nothing else on my mind but the ABC visit.

From the jetport we went to the site of the next morning's remote broadcast and walked through everything with the network people. Just in time for the six o'clock news (which I was field producing and directing from the same spot), we finished with ABC. We agreed we'd all meet the following morning around four o'clock and be on national TV with ABC's *World News This Morning* at 6:00 A.M. *Good Morning America* would start an hour later.

I did the 6:00 and 11:00 P.M. news work and helped pack all the remote equipment into our mobile truck. Just as I was about to leave for my hotel, someone announced that the staff wanted me to take them out for a drink. I looked at my watch—it was midnight. I had to be back in four hours but I was the only department head in Myrtle Beach, making me the only person with an expense account. I gave in to their urging and took the crew out for a couple of beers.

By 2:00 A.M. I was finally in my hotel room, watching the digital clock in the darkness, replaying the previous week and thinking about all that was yet to come. The pressure and exertion were becoming a bit much even for me. I finally dozed for a short while until the alarm jarred me from sleep at 3:30 A.M. I dragged myself into a hot steamy shower, psyching myself up for the national ABC remote and our station's own marathon weekend.

The GMA remote came and went, as did the special newscasts, local weather remotes, and parade and bikini contest. The broadcasts were all very successful and I was very satisfied that I had managed to coordinate it all. Late Saturday, I limped back home and packed for my next adventure. I was beginning to drag a bit from the fatigue.

The next morning, Sunday, June 4, at 6:40 A.M. I boarded a commuter flight from Florence to Charlotte. The previous week was now just a blur. I gulped down coffee and danish in the Charlotte airport and caught the 9:05 flight to Los Angeles.

That night, I was mingling with the stars at a cocktail reception. The food and drink spread was incredible, but I felt my eyes getting heavy. I decided it was time to head back to my room high in the luxurious Century Plaza Hotel for some long-overdue sleep. But wait—I hadn't exercised yet that day! So I returned to my room where I religiously donned my shorts and running shoes. After that, I ran up and down the fire stairs for about twenty minutes, making sure I got my daily dose of exercise. I'm sure sleep came quickly that night, no matter what was on my mind.

Los Angeles was a great week for me. I got to meet my favorite TV star, Dana Delany of China Beach. We posed for a picture together. I asked her if she was a Dodger fan—there was a home game tomorrow. She asked me if I was married. That took care of that!

The next day, with the California presidential primary just around the corner, we were surprised during a meeting with ABC

News President Roone Arledge. The three remaining presidential candidates—George Bush, Jesse Jackson, and Michael Dukakis—all made their way to the stage. ABC News anchor Peter Jennings moderated the impromptu discussion. It was great, a private presidential debate just for us. I wanted to call everyone back home and tell them what was happening.

When the meeting adjourned, most of the people in the audience headed for the hallway and the coffee pots. I rushed for the stage. Jennings was just coming down from the risers, bearing an expression I knew well. It was the I-just-came-off-a-performance-and-want-someone's-opinion look.

"How did it look?" he asked. He was talking to *me.*

"Umm, great," I stammered. "I mean, just fine. It went really well. We were all surprised and really impressed."

Jennings's mind must have been racing. He glanced at his watch. In the TV business, timing is everything, and I'm sure if Jennings had gone over his time limit by even a minute or two, he was upset with himself.

"But didn't we seem to go a little long?" he asked, in his slightly accented tone.

"Long?" I wasn't prepared to offer criticism to America's number-one anchor. "No, it wasn't long. One of those three men will be the next President. It couldn't have gone too long. It was just right."

I was displaced from Jennings by Arledge, who had just seen the candidates out the door.

"How'd it look?" Jennings asked him, without making eye contact. He was again looking at his watch. "Did we go too long?"

I bumped into White House correspondent and self-proclaimed nasty boy Sam Donaldson and introduced myself. I rode up to my room on the elevator with the legendary David Brinkley. At a party that night, Spencer Christian called out to me from across the crowd. I felt as if I belonged, as if I were somebody. I loved the TV business, and even though I felt unusually tired during that week, my time in Los Angeles had turned out to be a fantasy come true.

3

BITTEN IN BAHAMA

"Ladies and gentlemen, from the flight deck . . . We've been cleared for our approach into Nassau. Current Nassau weather is overcast skies with light rain, temperature eighty-two, with light winds from the south. Sorry about the rain, folks, but we'll have you on the ground in about ten minutes." The pilot's final sentence was met by a collective sigh of disappointment from the passengers. None of them was flying to Nassau for the rain.

I thought of Hettie in the seat beside me. I wanted this vacation for her. She deserved it. I'd spent only one night in my own bed since returning from Los Angeles, and I would have just as readily enjoyed a few days off at home. But she knew I'd never do that. We had to get away, or I'd just keep on working. She'd seen so little of me these past weeks. Between *Good Morning America*, the Sun Fun Festival, and my trip to LA, I felt Hettie deserved better than overcast skies and light rain.

As we taxied toward the tiny terminal a few moments later, I studied the skies hopefully for signs of clearing.

The beautiful Bahamian sunshine did return the next day, and we spent a relaxing afternoon in the waters of Cable Beach. That night, we went to another nearby hotel for dinner. I didn't know it then, but my body was all but asking to be attacked by whatever bug might be in the air. I'd been run down, gone days without sleep, been through incalculable stress, still felt jet lag from my LA trip, and had weakened what immune resistance might have been remaining by spending the day in the sun. The last two weeks—indeed, the previous two years—had worn me thin beneath the

34

tough exterior I always showed. If there was a bug to be caught, my body would be a willing host.

We walked the half-mile or so to dinner that night and enjoyed the summer air. The only nuisances were an occasional crazy driver whizzing by too fast and too close and the buzzing of a few pesky mosquitos.

As we sat down to order our meal, Hettie noticed an ugly red welt on my left arm.

"Did you hit your arm on something?" she asked.

I looked closer at it and saw a tiny puncture wound.

"Mosquito bite," I told her, and we both remarked about how it was causing a strange reaction on my arm. The entire portion from my elbow to my hand was turning red and swelling up. It was beginning to hurt, too. I had never had an allergic reaction to any bee stings or bug bites, so this experience made an impression on us both, and would be recalled by Hettie nearly two years later.

There may never be a way to prove it scientifically, but after careful study of my medical records and other notes I've kept, I believe that at that very moment I was being infected with what would eventually be sought in laboratories across the country—a possible viral agent behind an illness called chronic fatigue syndrome (CFS), or chronic fatigue and immune dysfunction syndrome (CFIDS). Four years after that, certain members of the CFS/CFIDS population would receive a new label—"non-HIV AIDS," or idiopathic CD4+T-lymphocytopenia (ICL).

Regardless of whether I'm right about the mosquito bite's playing a role in my illness, just six weeks later, my body began to fall apart.

There's plenty of scientific proof of that.

4

THE FLU THAT DIDN'T GO AWAY

Among the many other things I was doing during the summer of 1988, I was also working toward my commercial pilot license. I'd been a private pilot since 1984, added my instrument rating in 1987, and eventually wanted to become a flight instructor in my "spare" time. The required next step was getting the commercial ticket.

I flew with my commercial instructor a couple of nights each week and early on Saturday or Sunday mornings. Working toward the commercial was—after four years of flying—finally making me feel comfortable in an airplane. I honed and tested my own abilities, and I was learning to do things with an airplane I had only seen others do. It was a joy and a pleasure to fly, and my confidence grew with each lesson. When I wasn't flying, I was reading aviation books or studying aircraft manuals, learning airplanes and their systems inside-out. I also studied for the FAA's written commercial test, which measured my knowledge about things I'd never use, such as the weight and balance computations for a Boeing 727, and scores of regulations that air carriers must live by.

Still, I committed the material to my photographic memory, and scored a near-perfect mark on the written exam. I was thoroughly enjoying my expedition into the world of professional aviation. As my television career seemed to be finally in the big leagues, so was my flying, and I could not have been happier about it.

A year or two earlier, I'd met up with an exceptional man who came to believe that my flying abilities might one day account for something more than just a hobby. He eventually sponsored much of my training. We became close friends, and set our sights on a $500,000 airplane called the Piper Malibu.

My friend has great vision, and while neither of us had the half-million dollars needed to buy the airplane, he never suggested that such a picayune detail would get between us and the Malibu. I knew he had some powerful friends of his own, so I just strapped myself in for the ride.

In that same summer of 1988, we decided that I should go to Vero Beach, Florida, home of Piper Aircraft, and attend Piper's Malibu School. Since the plane was a sophisticated model with a pressurized cabin, turbocharged engine, and state-of-the-art electronics, only a fool would try to fly one without first going to school to learn all about it. And graduating from the school was also a requirement of most insurance underwriters before they'd allow you to fly the sleek aircraft.

And so, in late July, just six weeks after returning from the Bahamas, Hettie and I packed the car for a week in Florida. We would stop on the way for a night in St. Augustine, as we'd done once before on a previous visit to Piper.

The night before we left, lying in bed, I noticed a slight tickle in the back of my throat. I'd never let sickness slow me down for a moment, so I ignored the sore throat and the slight fever that accompanied it, and we set off early the next morning for St. Augustine.

By the time we arrived, I was coughing horribly, and felt as if I were coming down with the flu. Even if I'd wanted to give in to the symptoms and head home, I couldn't. Malibu School was already paid for, and so were our reservations at one of Vero Beach's finest hotels.

That night in St. Augustine, I could hardly sleep for the incessant coughing, but in the morning we pressed on toward Vero Beach, dismissing my discomfort as a rare summer cold.

My condition worsened in Vero. My voice was too weak to speak most of the time during classroom sessions. I had to sleep propped up in a chair to keep from choking on the fluid that was collecting in my lungs. It was a miserable way to spend what was supposed to be a fun week, but I didn't let it stop me. I wanted to fly the Malibu. Nothing else mattered. I would graduate with high marks, period.

On Thursday, July 28, I graduated from both the classroom and flying portions of the school. So sick and weak I could hardly speak, I had qualified to fly the world's most sophisticated single-engine piston airplane. The pleasure of that accomplishment seemed to buoy my spirits, and the long drive home the next day passed uneventfully.

In the weeks that followed, I lived as normally as possible, but I found myself compensating for something I couldn't quite put my finger on. All my life, I'd taught myself to ignore physical symptoms and ailments. Just as I would do when I got the nails in my feet after Hurricane Hugo, I simply pressed on with what had to be done and worried about mending later.

I spent the last week of August 1988 doing both my promotion job and being the weathercaster. But for the first time since I'd taken on the weather job, I asked Bill Christian if I could come to work late on days after I had done the weather, rather than working from 8:00 A.M. to midnight.

That week took a toll on me as none before it ever had. Between the 6:00 and 11:00 P.M. news, I would come home and collapse onto the bed, lying there until the last possible minute before heading back to the studio. Maybe I was pushing myself too hard, I remember thinking. After all, I was nearly thirty.

Another significant event happened about the same time. Hettie and I were wrestling on our bed one Saturday morning. She surprised me with a quick reversal and sent me flying, and I hit the base of my skull against the molding around the bottom of our nightstand. I suffered a severe concussion, and spent a week in a semi-dazed state. Yes, I told the doctors, I know who the president is, but I don't feel like me. I had trouble thinking at times, and just gave up doing paperwork by the time the afternoons arrived. Bill kept trying to send me home from work. Once he found me wandering the halls, having forgotten where I was heading.

I now know the significance of a head injury in the eventual course of my illness, and can boil it down to a simple sentence.

Once the brain suffers an injury, it's much more susceptible to damage from other illness. The concussion became something of a joke, but it would later serve to confuse my diagnosis and, I am certain, pave the way for the forthcoming CFS viral attack on my brain. The virus that I suspect had entered my body two months earlier in the Bahamas now had a clear path to my brain.

Through the fog of my concussion, through the demands of my job, through the joyous rigors of flight training, I knew something wasn't right with my body. It just wouldn't do what I wanted it to do. This was something new to me, something that I didn't want to admit. In addition to what now appears to have been the further manifestation of my illness, I was beginning to deal with something else equally insidious, and perhaps even more deadly in the long run: denial.

I spent September 2 taking the practical portion of the commercial pilot test. By the end of the day, the examiner was typing out my new commercial pilot certificate. I was now able to get paid for flying.

This was not my ultimate goal at all. The commercial license meant that I was simply one step closer to earning an instructor's rating and being able to teach others what had become one of my life's joys. I hastily ordered an expensive set of videotapes that would help prepare me for the instructor written exam. Strangely, though, when they arrived I found I didn't have the energy to watch them after work, and when I did finally force myself to put a tape into the VCR, I had a hard time concentrating on the material. I never finished that first tape, and I'm sure that even today it is still at exactly the point it was when I popped it out of my VCR.

I would go on to log just one paid flying job, a simple trip for a local photographer. I made twenty-five dollars, but I wasn't into flying for the money, and I had already invested more than fifteen thousand dollars in my pursuit of aviation.

The instructor exam tapes remain untouched on my bookshelf, and I never came to realize my dream of teaching others to fly. I didn't know it at the time, but my own days in airplanes were drawing to a close. It would still be more than a year before I understood why.

I continued to struggle along as the number-two weathercaster, making it through a three-day stint in September and an entire week in October. Instead of a joy, each on-air experience became like pushing a boulder uphill. I leaned wearily against the weather set until seconds before the director gave me my cue, and then I would turn on the smile for three or four minutes until my segment had passed. Many times, I slumped to the ground or against a set riser the moment I was off the air.

On October 15, Hettie and I took off on our annual pilgrimage to Kennebunkport, Maine. A TV contact in Boston, Jack King, had been inviting us to his Maine home each fall to see the leaves change, and Hettie and I always jumped at the chance. Kennebunkport, especially in the fall, is beautiful, and the Kings are great hosts. I remember packing my running shoes, telling myself I'd been too busy to work out lately, and that I'd get back into the swing of things in the cool, crisp Maine air.

On Sunday, October 16, I laced up the shoes and set off into the chilly morning at Goose Rocks Beach, just north of Kennebunkport. I was full of optimism and denial.

I made it about two hundred yards before I had to turn back.

November brought our station's ratings period, and somehow I made it through. "Sweeps," as they are called, come four times each year, and they're brutal on a promotion director. Other than sweeps, I don't imagine I did much of anything worth writing down.

December 2 was the last time I piloted an aircraft and felt as if I knew what I was doing 100 percent of the time. I noticed I was having good weeks and bad weeks—this one was going well. Two local football teams had made it to the state final that night, and the only way to get the video back for the 11 P.M. news was by airplane. It was a bitter cold night, which made for crystal clear skies. On the return trip, we were slightly ahead of schedule, and I climbed to more than a mile high. We were over the center of South Carolina, and could see forever in every direction. It was as if God Himself knew I was nearing the horrible hiatus in my flying career, and He had shined up the heavens for one last display.

Hettie and Richard Perdue, the same photographer who would be with me in Hugo, were along for the ride. It was glorious. There were stars everywhere, billions of them. And on the ground, tiny lights twinkled up at us. The Carolina countryside was already decked out for the holidays.

Hettie and I dropped Richard off at the Florence airport and returned the airplane to its home in Sumter, about forty miles away. By the time the landing gear chirped onto Runway 22, our spirits were high, but our energy was sagging.

When we finally arrived home at around eleven o'clock, we found sad news on the answering machine. My grandfather, hospitalized earlier in the week for a routine illness, had died at about the same time we were a mile high over the state. I was saddened at the news, but I knew we couldn't mourn. My admired grandfather had lived a full and wonderful life. And I knew in my heart the view of the heavens he had that night was much more spectacular than even ours had been.

We flew to Pennsylvania the following day, and twenty-four hours after that our family gathered for my grandpa's funeral. While on that trip, I promised my cousin I'd come to Washington, D.C., soon to visit her and her family. I never found the energy to keep my promise.

When we returned from the funeral trip, I remember heading to the fitness club to try again to hit the running track.

"This just isn't *right*," I told Hettie after I'd returned, exhausted without making it a half-mile. "I'm not even thirty years old!"

Oh, well, I told myself, I'd been under a lot of stress lately. Some rest over the holidays would do me well. It might also break that nagging fever that was dogging me, and help me to reclaim a decent night's sleep. Lately, I'd wake up after an hour or two, drenched in sweat yet chilled to the bone.

I'm just under a lot of pressure, I kept telling myself. Things would get better. They always did.

5

REAL MEN DON'T GET SICK

In the coming weeks, I quietly started avoiding the fitness club and ordered a stair-climber exercise machine from L. L. Bean. I could have bought the same piece of equipment locally (and cheaper), but in the back of my mind was Bean's "no questions asked" return policy. After the stair-climber was delivered and Hettie had assembled it, I tried it about a half-dozen times; only once did I last more than a minute or two. Only a few months earlier, I had run up and down the stairs at the Century Plaza Hotel after a twenty-hour day. The stair-climber was shunted to a back room, and soon after we shipped it back to Bean's.

Hettie and I were always aware of my demanding schedule and how difficult I always found it to take time off. My vacation weeks were never used up by year's end, and we usually let the excess pass without a mention. But this year, I was feeling guilty that I hadn't even taken Hettie to dinner or a movie lately. In an attempt to make up for this, I tried to squeeze in a quick Florida vacation between Christmas and New Year's.

The effort of getting everything finished in my one-man department drained me as Hettie packed our bags. I remember little about the trip itself except thinking it was much too little, far too late, and the drive nearly killed me. I'd been feeling ill for months, and a few days' vacation didn't change that.

The new year brought the effort of a major fundraiser set for George Bush's inauguration night, January 20, 1989. Our television station was helping the local Literacy Council raise money to combat illiteracy, a favorite cause for the soon-to-be First Lady, Barbara

Bush. Mrs. Bush sent me a lovely letter which was read at our event at the same moment she and her husband were attending inaugural balls throughout Washington. Our own event, which we called "The Inaugural Ball for Literacy," helped raise more than $10,000 in just one evening. I had worked on the project since August, and when the celebrities and management from our station showed up that night, they were impressed with my accomplishments. As I look back on the event, I think that night was the last time ever that the "party" side of Tim was seen by anyone. I know that I attended several awards banquets and other affairs in my remaining time with WPDE, but I was always the last to arrive and the first to leave. This night, however, I donned my brand new tuxedo and enjoyed the festivities. Photographs of the event, though, suggest that I didn't work the crowd as I usually did; they show me sitting quietly at our company table. Still, my signature smile is in those photos, and though I was definitely on a downhill slide, I'd give anything today to slip on that tux and go back to that evening. Though I would continue working for more than two years after that night, I have never since felt that carefree attitude you can see in those photos. The tuxedo hangs in the back of my closet, having been out only once since then. In some ways, the Inaugural Ball for Literacy was my going-away party.

Only days after the ball, the February sweeps loomed ominously. I ached for relief, and there was none in sight.

Sleep had become nearly impossible. Dreams, complete with strange colors and near-hallucinations, haunted what rest I could find. The night sweats worsened. I moved from our bedroom to the living room sofa so my tossing wouldn't disturb Hettie.

Some mornings, I wasn't able to drag myself to work until ten o'clock, and I really had no excuse to offer. Still, my boss stuck with me, though I was told some others were carefully watching my new habits. That angered me, because no one was especially mindful when I was working seven-day weeks, or when I worked late while the rest of the managers were out enjoying happy hour.

Throughout all of this, though it may seem incongruous, I maintained a relatively fair degree of functioning and sociability. I remained the station's chief idea man, I still cranked out more than a hundred new promo spots each week, and my work continued to take top honors at local awards competitions. See, I kept telling myself, *there's nothing wrong with you. You can still do it all.*

But then something unusual started happening that I couldn't hide from myself or others. My near-perfect memory seemed to disappear, especially when I was extremely fatigued. My boss called the expression that accompanied my confusion the "concussion look," a reference to my confused state of mind after that incident the year before, and we'd all have a laugh about my wife's throwing me off the bed.

By spring, the concussion look was appearing two or three times a week, usually late in the afternoon. Though the doctors who had treated me at the time of my concussion said the mental problems would clear up in a few days, I still blamed these new episodes on that accident.

"This is serious," our news anchor told me privately. "You're starting to repeat yourself all the time. People are noticing. I'm worried about you."

"I'm just so busy that I'm forgetting stuff," I told her. I didn't bring up the swollen glands, the unbearable headaches that no medicine could help, and the pain in my joints which was so intense that I'd often wrap bandages around my wrists and ankles at night to keep them from moving. I was trying to look and act like the old Tim. Everything was just fine. That was what I wanted everyone, especially myself, to believe.

I flew an airplane two or three times that spring, but never felt totally comfortable doing it. I could still make the airplane go where I wanted it to, but things sometimes got jumbled, and I had a hard time sorting them out. Fortunately, the flights were local photography flights for our news department in perfect weather, and no one was ever in jeopardy.

On March 30, my father was in a serious automobile accident in Pennsylvania. I flew there just a few hours later, rented a car, and drove three hours to the tiny hospital that was trying to keep him alive. During the drive, a chilling thought hit me: I couldn't remember what kind of plane I had flown up on. Sure, my thoughts were with my father, but I always knew what kind of plane I was in. *Always*. When I flew on a commercial jet, I always noted when the pilots changed power settings on the engines, when the flaps and slats were deployed, when the landing gear were dropped. I always paid attention to those things, and I *certainly* knew what kind of plane I flew on. Ask any recreational pilot; a commercial airline flight is a savored experience.

The hair on my neck stood up. I had no memory of the flight at all. Somehow, I'd just rented a Pontiac in Pittsburgh and was driving on the Pennsylvania Turnpike. It was shock, I told myself—the shock of my father's accident had blocked my memory. Were it not for that, I'd know everything about the trip from Florence to Pittsburgh. But the fact was that I didn't yet know about my father's near-fatal injuries. Sure, I was concerned about him, but I was really making the trip as a show of support for my mother. My mind wasn't occupied by thoughts of my father's possible death. I wasn't in any state of shock. I simply could not remember the flight.

My father was transferred to a major trauma center the next day. His condition was critical and deteriorating when we transferred him via air ambulance. Three days later, the doctors felt that my dad was out of the woods; he would recover. Bowing to the mounting demands back at the television station, I flew home the next day. This time I forced myself to remember: I flew on a Boeing 737.

The trip to Pennsylvania had brought another startling event, every bit as disquieting as my memory lapse. On the second night I was there, while staying at my brother's home, I passed out while on my way to the bathroom in the middle of the night. I awakened some minutes later lying flat on my face, with the most terrible head pain I had ever experienced. I had black eyes and a sore nose for days, but more than that, I was actually frightened by what happened. I had headed to the bathroom, and ended up unconscious.

I had three more loss-of-consciousness experiences in the next few months, and each time I ended up bruised and scared. I was now having objective symptoms—there was no need to interpret what these events meant, as one might with a jumbled memory.

Without cause or warning, I was passing out. That meant something. I couldn't be imagining these experiences. I had the bruises to prove they happened, and someone else usually heard me fall and found me.

By June, the evidence of my memory problems was overwhelming. I let my anchorwoman friend make me an appointment with one of her doctors. I hated going to the doctor's office. After all, I had never really been sick in my life. Admitting to being ill would be a sign of weakness. Still, my friend's fears about me were beginning to rub off on me. I kept the appointment.

"Memory problems are indicative of many things," the doctor began. "Most likely, you're just busy, and like a computer disk, you can store only so much information."

I liked his explanation so far.

"Or it could be something else," he said coldly. "Maybe a thyroid problem, maybe MS, maybe even a brain tumor. Or this could have something to do with your concussion. Let's schedule you for some tests."

Why couldn't he have stopped with the computer disk?

That explanation made sense to me. It was June 13, just one week after another *Good Morning America* weather remote in Myrtle Beach, another Sun Fun Festival, another parade and bikini contest, another series of local news and weather remotes, and another telethon weekend. I didn't mention the mounting list of other symptoms to the doctor. Looking back, though, I fault him more than me for not delving deeper. I presented with severe memory dysfunction at the age of thirty. He should have asked if anything else was wrong! Then I probably would have remembered the other things. No wonder I hated going to doctors. Your life could be falling apart, and you'd have two-and-a-half minutes to explain it all.

June 27 found me at the nearest hospital with an MRI machine, beginning the series of tests ordered by Dr. Computer Disk. MRI—magnetic resonance imaging—is the state-of-the-art way to take pictures of the brain. Dr. Disk had ordered this test, along with an electroencephalogram (EEG) and a thyroid function test.

My denial instinct was so strong that I almost didn't show up for the outpatient procedure. If something was seriously wrong, I thought, what good would it do me to know? And if I were merely an overloaded computer disk, why go to all this fuss? But my memory problems were beginning to handicap my work and every other part of my life. And there were the times that I had passed out . . .

"Name?" the compassionless receptionist asked, staring straight down at her computer.

"Timothy P. Kenny. K-E-N-N-Y."

"Age?"

"Thirty."

I'd turned thirty back in March, but had never been asked my age since then and had never spoken the number in that context. I suddenly felt old.

A short time later, wearing only a one-size-doesn't-fit-all hospital gown, I was flat on my back on a table, about to be slid into the multimillion-dollar MRI machine. A plastic helmet would hold my head in place. The technician put foam plugs into my ears to help deaden the loud clicking I was told to expect.

"Are you claustrophobic?" someone asked.

As the motorized slab moved me into the MRI tube, I thought of James Bond strapped down on some conveyor belt, headed toward death. Was that what awaited me? Would these tests show something awful growing inside my head? I acknowledged the possibility, and then drifted off to sleep despite the loud magnetic clicking of the MRI. It was the first daytime nap I'd been able to grab in more than a year. Perhaps the clicking sounds hypnotized me, or perhaps I just took rest and refuge in the belief that this giant machine would be able to figure out my problem.

But if the machine figured it out, no one called to tell me.

One day passed, then another. The doctor had promised he'd call with the results. The news must be bad, I reasoned, and my friend who had referred me to Dr. Disk didn't disagree with me. By now, I freely admitted to my memory lapses, and suggested that perhaps I'd misunderstood the doctor's promise to inform me of the test results.

"At least, I *think* he said he'd call," I told my friend.

Finally, on the third day of pins-and-needles waiting, we got Dr. Disk's nurse to release the results over the phone. Everything was negative; the tests found nothing unusual. My friend and I rejoiced at the news, but it really didn't help. I had hoped to have some quick diagnosis of my condition. Instead, I was left with the nagging question of what was wrong with me.

The doctor had told me that he'd follow up the tests with a phone call and another visit, even if the results were negative. "We'll try some other things, in that case," he had said. "Gotta rule out MS and all that."

I never heard from Dr. Disk again.

A few days after I learned the test results, my boss and friend Bill Christian, the station's general manager, called me and another department head into the conference room. He was considering major changes in the news department, perhaps firing some people whom I cared about. I felt he was missing the point—instead of changing people, he needed to change attitudes and ideas. But I never disagreed with him in front of another person, so I followed him to his office after the meeting.

"You don't need new anchors," I told him. "You need new ideas. You need that department to quit worrying about what they think the competition is doing, and start producing newscasts that people will switch to." Such thinking is a typical trap into which number-two television stations fall—copying the number-one station instead of trying to come up with a totally different and superior product. Bill asked me to continue, and I began spouting ideas from the top of my aching head.

The next morning, he called me into his office. "I stayed awake last night thinking about what you said," he said flatly. (At least I wasn't the only one losing sleep!) "Everything you said made sense," he continued, pushing his chair back from the desk like bosses do to punctuate a major transition.

"Aw, hell," he began in a different tone. "Let me just say it. I want you to be my new news director. You're the one who's making the most sense around here."

It was high praise for a guy whose computer disk wasn't holding up under the strain of a one-man department. How could I take on the responsibility for the station's largest, most expensive, most visible entity in this condition? I didn't even know what my condition was. Yet the coach was asking me to pitch the big game. How could I say no?

After I voiced my concerns and asked a few questions, Bill said, "I'll be away until after the Fourth of July. Have your answer ready then. And by the way," he continued quietly, "I've found the money for the major news expansion you've always wanted us to have."

For as long as Bill and I had worked together, I'd been pushing for a greater presence along the coast in Myrtle Beach, more people, more equipment, and a noon newscast. Now he was offering to give me a chance to make it all happen. "Sleep on it," he said.

I wish I could have slept on his offer. I wish I just could have *slept*. I hadn't gone into his office that day to get the news director's job. No one moved from promotion to news. The idea hadn't even crossed my mind. I did have years of news experience, and had even produced many of our news specials. Still, there would be people at the station who would believe I had jockeyed for the job and wanted to displace the guy who now had it. Back-stabbing is not uncommon in the television industry. The current news director was a friend of mine, a flying buddy. Maybe I didn't agree with everything he did to run his department, but I didn't want him to lose his job. And I certainly didn't want to be the one to take it from him. (This man and I remain friends today.)

Bill returned on July 5, and I shuffled reluctantly toward his office. "Well?" he began.

His question hung in the air. We were alone in the office, the door closed.

"I don't want Bob to lose his job," I said.

"He'll stay on as anchor. I'll even give him a raise," Bill said, staring at me with a wry smile. "Look," he continued, "I'm going to get a new news director one way or the other. You're just my first choice."

The coach was making a pitching change, signaling for me to come in and save the game. To heck with all my weird symptoms that made no sense. Forget about my forgetfulness. If the coach wanted me to pitch, I'd pitch.

He named a salary, and we shook hands on the deal.

My first day on the new job, I sent a memo to the controller giving myself a minor pay cut. Officially a part of the news department now, I didn't think it was proper that I should get paid for the times I filled in as weathercaster. I also handed out three overdue raises that afternoon. My third day on the job, I fired someone for the first time in my life. Being a boss had its rewards and its painful experiences. Still, I was beginning to feel I'd been destined for this job since I first knocked on WPDE's door six years earlier.

Two weeks later, Bill and his wife, Hettie and myself, and another department head were on beautiful Hilton Head Island for the annual meeting of the South Carolina Broadcasters' Association. Attending that meeting was my first perk as news director. Bill called the mixed business/pleasure trip payback for "hell week"—the Sun Fun Festival and *Good Morning America* remotes.

Our second night there, something strange happened. Passing through the hotel lobby, I walked right into a heavy, five-foot sign that pointed toward the lounge. The force of the collision knocked the sign over, and it fell with an incredible clangor, smashing my left foot. Although I laughed along with the rest of our group, this was no mere act of clumsiness—*I simply hadn't seen the sign.*

The night manager rushed over and acted as if I were a barroom drunk. He looked at me with disgust, and mumbled something about my drinking to one of his assistants. Drinking? The glass I'd been carrying contained ice water. I was stone sober.

I spent several hours at Hilton Head hospital the next morning having my foot x-rayed, and my grossly swollen foot kept me reclining by the pool for the rest of the trip. I was also afraid of what else I might run into if I walked around.

In the coming weeks, I poured myself into my new job, even handling my old job until a replacement was found. I began to interview applicants for the news expansion—we would be adding a noon newscast and expanding our morning news as soon as I had the people and plan in place. The expansion, set for August 14, remained a secret, and I raced against the deadline despite my worsening physical and cognitive symptoms.

On August 14, we kicked off the market's first noon newscast, taking the competition by surprise. My staff had grown from sixteen to twenty-two, and I still had some positions left to fill. I had come a long way from running a one-person department to being on the leading edge of our station's expansion. Yet despite this fantasy-come-true, I sensed I was living on borrowed time.

A month after we initiated our noon news program, I was in Kansas City for the Radio and Television News Directors' Association convention that I mentioned at the beginning of this book. A week after that, Hurricane Hugo smashed into South Carolina, changing our state and our lives forever.

Still reeling from Hugo, knowing I was ready to drop in my tracks, Hettie and I went ahead with our annual Kennebunkport trip in mid-October 1989. (Though we would make the airline reservations again a year later, I would by then be too sick to make the trip, and Hettie went with my mother, instead.) On this visit, the Kings were again superb hosts, and the respite and lobster seemed to perk me up. I was thankful to get away from all the hurricane damage. The "concussion look" stayed away while we were in Maine, but I remember my joints hurting terribly, and I recall desperately seeking relief through whatever over-the-counter medicines I could find. The horrible pain was a disappointing distraction during what was to be my last vacation in Maine.

Soon after I returned to South Carolina, I demoted myself from being backup weathercaster, telling everyone my new job was just too demanding to allow this distraction. For me, not being able to appear on-air was a psychological blow, but there was no way I could maintain the rigors of management and go on the air as well.

Looking back, one of the main reasons I demoted myself was exactly the same reason I might have done the same thing with one of my staff: I simply wasn't dependable anymore. I needed a weathercaster I could count on, and I was no longer that person.

Some days, I could barely make it to the office. I hastily trained someone else for the job, and he was excited to have the chance.

Late one afternoon near Christmas, I collapsed to the floor of my office with the worst chest pain I had ever experienced. My FAA physical exams had involved cardiac stress tests and regular EKGs, and I'd always been found to be in great cardiovascular shape. Yet when this horrible pain struck, I thought of my father and the heart attack he had in his early thirties. I crawled to the sofa along my office wall where Bill Christian found me a short time later. He called Hettie and made her promise that she'd take me directly to the hospital.

Hospital emergency rooms tend to move slowly, but a patient with severe chest pains gets prompt attention. The doctor who gave me a hasty exam quickly ordered an EKG. The results were entirely normal. There was no explanation for my sudden severe chest pain. Blood tests revealed no telltale enzymes pointing to a heart attack, and all the other tests failed to illuminate a cause. The doctor told me that stress may have caused the pain, or possibly a serious stomach ailment was to blame.

When he referred me for a follow-up visit with my local physician, I didn't tell him that this presented something of a problem—I didn't *have* a local physician! There was Dr. Disk, but I wasn't going back to him. In my denial and my zeal to keep performing TV miracles, I hadn't thought I needed a local physician.

I still thought I'd never been sick a day in my life.

6

MIND FOG

On Christmas Eve, 1989, a surprise weather system brought our area of South Carolina its first white Christmas in more than 150 years. Throughout the region, everyone marveled at this unusual event. My holiday outing was making my way outside, taking a photograph of our house blanketed in snow, and stumbling back to the sofa. A week later, I rang in the New Year lying quietly in bed.

By now, I was convinced that *something* was wrong with me. Though I had put off seeing a physician after my emergency treatment at the hospital before Christmas, I decided I'd better find someone to check me out. I needed to get some answers.

Since I didn't have a family doctor, I went to the physician who'd administered my flight physicals. After a two-minute exam and a little aviation talk, he ordered some tests to see if there was anything wrong with my stomach. Since this doctor approved my aviation medical certificate, I didn't tell him about the horrible chest pains I'd had only a couple of weeks earlier. I only mentioned that I'd been having some slight "discomfort" in the area of my stomach.

On January 8, I was back in this doctor's waiting room to discuss the results of my tests. I sat for more than two hours in the outer office. I was furious. Something was wrong with me! Modern medicine should have figured this out by now. Besides, I had work to do!

Finally, a nurse called me in. She took me to an examining room, recorded my blood pressure and weight, and shoved a thermometer into my mouth.

"When do I get to see the doctor?" I asked, through teeth clenched around the thermometer. "He's two hours late already."

The nurse never looked at me. "The doctor is quite busy," she said, taking my pulse.

"When will he get to me?" I insisted.

She looked perturbed. "I don't know, probably within an hour," she offered grudgingly.

She was glaring now. Imagine the nerve of me, wanting some respect!

I'd had enough. Another hour of waiting, only to get two-and-a-half minutes with this guy? I had little patience for illness, and even less patience for doctors who kept me waiting only to tell me they had no answers.

"Look, let's just forget it," I said, jerking the thermometer out of my mouth. "Just look at my file. I had an upper GI test done last week. Are the results in?"

The nurse huffed, but slowly opened my file and studied it for a moment. "Your tests were normal."

"Then I'm outta here," I said. I wasn't going to wait three hours to see somebody who couldn't tell me what was wrong with me. I could imagine hearing the stress lecture again, or maybe this guy even knew the computer disk analogy. I knew it wasn't stress—I thrived on stress, ever since . . . *when?* I used to live for it, almost tempt it.

I just couldn't bear the thought of another doctor letting me down. Doctors, I had believed, were supposed to have answers. Why weren't they giving me any?

With the chest pains now a memory and another battery of tests turning up nothing, I began to consider for the first time that something might actually be wrong with my overall health, not just whatever part hurt or wasn't working well on a particular day. I tried in vain to describe for Hettie the feeling that accompanied the concussion look. I'd changed the name to "the helmet," because when it came I always felt that there was a giant lead helmet on my head. The helmet would slow down my thinking, get in the way of my memory, make me say the wrong words, and sometimes cause me to burst out in rage.

"The helmet," I kept saying, trying to make her understand. That description was still lacking. I was a journalist, yet I couldn't come up with the words to describe what was happening to me.

But then I learned that someone else already had.

I was driving home for lunch one afternoon in February when I tuned the radio to hear commentator Paul Harvey. Among his stories that day was a report about a group of scientists meeting in Los Angeles to discuss an illness some called the "yuppie flu." Among its symptoms, Harvey noted, were extreme fatigue, severe headaches, muscle pain, weakness—

I wasn't taking him very seriously. He said the malady was officially called chronic fatigue syndrome, which sounded like lawyer-talk for burnout.

—and mind fog.

I'll never forget the exact spot where I was on the highway when I heard that term. *That was it!* That was the concussion look, the helmet! *Mind fog* was the term I'd been searching for.

I pulled off at the next gas station to buy a *USA Today*. This "yuppie flu" sounded like the kind of story that paper would jump on. I didn't have to look far—the story, by Kim Painter, was on page one.

Unraveling Mystery of "Yuppie Flu"

Many scientists now strongly suspect chronic fatigue syndrome—once despairingly dubbed "yuppie flu"—is a complex disorder of the immune system and brain, rather than a simple viral disease. Lab findings and symptoms—which can include constant recurring fatigue, mental fogginess, flu-like symptoms, allergies and a pronounced intolerance for exercise—indicate patients have overactive immune systems, says Dr. Paul Cheney of Charlotte, N.C., among experts meeting in Los Angeles over the weekend.

"It's really the opposite of AIDS. We're looking at patients whose immune systems are up-regulated."

The term *mental fogginess* jumped out at me, jarring me as Paul Harvey's words had. The other symptoms fit as well. Maybe I had stumbled onto something. How could anyone else know about the helmet, the concussion look, the mind fog, unless he was talking about the same thing I had?

Skimming the opening paragraphs of the USA *Today* story again the moment I got home, something else struck me. Painter had quoted a doctor from Charlotte, North Carolina, just over two hours from my home. I dropped the newspaper and reached for the telephone, dialing directory assistance for area code 704.

"Dr. Paul Cheney, please," I asked the operator, and quickly copied the number.

When I dialed, the receptionist told me that Dr. Cheney no longer practiced at that location. Did she have another number for him? Yes, she did, and I copied it down.

"One more thing," I asked. "What is his specialty?"

"Chronic Epstein-Barr virus," the woman told me, though I now know her information was somewhat out of date.

I scribbled that on a piece of paper, not knowing I'd just begun the long and frustrating pursuit of a proper diagnosis and an effective treatment for what was wrong with me.

7

OFF TO SEE THE "WIZARD"

Although it was just noon, I knew that the appearance of Painter's front-page story in *USA Today* would probably mean that Dr. Cheney's office was being swamped with phone calls. Several busy signals later, I finally got Cheney's receptionist on the line.

"I'll bet you're getting lots of calls because of the newspaper article," I said, trying to sound nonchalant. I was calling upon my best acting ability. I really felt that Cheney, being so close to me and practically falling into my lap out of the blue, was something of a lifeline, but I didn't want to sound desperate.

"Whew!" the receptionist said, "It's been crazy all morning." Then she rattled off a list of cities from which she'd received calls in the last hour alone. The list sounded like the index of the *Exxon Travel Guide*. People from *everywhere* were calling this doctor.

I introduced myself, mentioned my occupation as a television news manager, and then asked the $64,000 question. "I was wondering if I could get an appointment with Dr. Cheney."

"Let's see," she said, and I could hear her flipping through the pages of the appointment book. I held my breath. Tomorrow wouldn't be soon enough.

"His next initial office visit is Thursday, June 21, at ten o'clock. But first I'll have to send you a questionnaire."

June? That was four months away. My heart sank, but I tried to sound reasonably composed.

"Okay, put me down for that," I agreed. At least it was a place to start. I could work on getting the appointment moved up later.

"But you have to fill out a twelve-page questionnaire before

Dr. Cheney can see you," the receptionist said. "He's heavily involved in research, and he gets calls from patients all over the world, and ..."

"Okay, I can do that," I injected quickly. I was sure my story was right up his alley. There was no question in my mind. "I'll give you my Federal Express account number. That way I can get the questionnaire tomorrow."

I couldn't wait for Bill Christian to get back from lunch. Being my boss, Bill held the power to replace me in a minute. But more than a boss, Bill was a very understanding friend. We had talked a lot about the helmet, and he was concerned for me because of my other problems. His actions on the day of my chest pains had proved to me that Bill was in my corner when I felt few others were.

"Ever hear of the Epstein-Barr virus?" I asked him. I had already forgotten the more current term *chronic fatigue syndrome*, remembering only *mind fog* and *Epstein-Barr*.

"Sure," he said, much to my surprise. "My old roommate's wife has it. She used to be a dancer. Now she can hardly do anything. I think she's gotten a little better lately, though."

I told Bill about the doctor in Charlotte, and showed him the *USA Today* article.

"Go for it," he encouraged me.

While talking to Bill, I attached a nickname to this Dr. Cheney in Charlotte, calling him "the Wizard." I wasn't foolish or desperate enough to think Cheney might possess magical powers; rather, I felt like the scarecrow in *The Wizard of Oz*—"if I only had a brain." If only I could see Cheney, I could get my brain back. I *had* to see the Wizard, I told Bill, and he agreed.

When the questionnaire arrived the next day, I immediately filled it out and returned it with a letter requesting an appointment as soon as possible. Acting as if I'd forgotten about June 21, I said Friday, March 2, would suit me just fine. There was no harm in trying to move up the date.

I was more convinced than ever that I was now on the right track. The old me kicked in—I had something to shoot for now,

the impossible to pull off. Because of a radio broadcast and a newspaper article, I had found someone who might be able to help me
put my life back together. June 21 was a long way off, but I'd find a
way to change that, too. At least for now I was making some
progress.

The night after I had spoken with Dr. Cheney's receptionist,
Hettie and I went to the library to research the Epstein-Barr virus.
We found very little in the medical books, although we learned
that the virus, part of the herpes family, appeared to be the agent
that caused mononucleosis. There were estimates that as much as
ninety percent of the U.S. adult population had been exposed to
it.

I was disappointed. I'd expected the medical encyclopedias to
be filled with articles about this ailment, chronic Epstein-Barr
virus, or maybe that other thing—what was it called?—chronic
fatigue syndrome. But even the latest encyclopedias reported nothing. Had I checked mainstream magazines and newspapers, I would
have found that Epstein-Barr and CFS were getting plenty of coverage—not from the medical community, but from the lay media.
Again, I'd made the mistake of looking to the medical establishment for answers. I went home from the library much as I had gone
home from earlier doctor's appointments—without answers and
full of disappointment.

What the media was reporting was that the disease came to
national attention during 1984 when two doctors in Incline
Village, Nevada, discovered a group of about two hundred patients
with the same symptoms that I'd been having. The patients didn't
get better, and a reluctant U.S. Centers for Disease Control (CDC)
was called in to investigate. The government's early and impotent
conclusion: Nothing significant was going on; perhaps the patients
were depressed, or maybe it was just a simple bug of some sort.
When I finally read about the Incline Village outbreak, I came
across the names of the two young doctors who'd called in the government's investigators—Daniel Peterson and Paul Cheney.

Cheney, it turned out, was nearly run out of town by his claims
that the illness was real and that it had some sort of organic basis.

He claimed that the outbreak was, in fact, a local epidemic. But Incline Village is a resort town on Lake Tahoe, and businesspeople and community leaders in resort towns don't take kindly to some young doctor even thinking the word *epidemic*. Cheney and his family eventually took refuge in Charlotte, and I suspect the final weeks in Nevada might have been difficult.

As an internal medicine specialist at the Nalle Clinic in Charlotte, Dr. Cheney began to come across patients with the same symptoms he'd seen in Nevada. Other patients from around the country had heard of him and sought him out. Cheney—far from being a quack or someone taken with fads—turned out to be one of only a few physicians who were taking these patients and their complaints seriously in the late 1980s. Back then he was viewed by many of his peers as an outcast; today, he is in demand at medical conventions around the world.

By January 1990, just over a month before I had heard of him, Cheney had opened his own practice. He was now treating and researching CFS full-time. I had no idea then how much courage that move must have taken. Even today many physicians in the Charlotte area and around the world distrust him. Others, I believe, resent that Cheney has achieved a worldwide reputation researching what history may show to be one of the fastest-spreading epidemics of its kind. Though it will always be overshadowed by AIDS, CFS is often called—even now by the medical establishment and government that earlier shunned it—"the disease of the '90s." And no matter how much flack he took in the early days, no one can deny today that Paul Cheney was one of the first to spot this unfolding epidemic and one of the first to sound the alarm.

After shipping the questionnaire back to Dr. Cheney's office, I impatiently waited a couple of days before calling. The receptionist remembered me.

"Did he get a chance to review my questionnaire?" I asked.

"It's right here," she answered, and I heard some papers rustling.

"What did he say?" I wanted to know.

"He wrote 'interesting' on it," she replied.

"Interesting." What did that mean?

"Will he *see me*?" I asked.

"Thursday, June 21, 10 A.M.," she answered evenly.

My mind raced. What card could I play to get what I wanted? I couldn't take *no* for an answer, but I couldn't alienate her.

"Okay, okay," I stalled. "June 21. Fine. But does he have a waiting list?"

"About three pages long," she answered quickly.

Strike two. I had to think of something *now*. "The first time we talked, you said he had patients from all over the country, right?"

"Really from all over the world," she responded. I could hear the pride.

"Okay . . . so most of these people fly in, right?" I asked.

"Most of them do fly in," the receptionist agreed.

"So if there's a cancellation . . . like a *last-minute* cancellation . . . then someone on the waiting list might need at least two days to book a flight, right?"

"Sure," she said. "Sometimes you need to book two weeks ahead to get the best fare."

"All right, here's the deal," I went on, as if *I* were the one offering hope to *them*. "I'm two hours away, maybe a little more. I'll keep my car gassed up every day. If you get a last-minute cancellation, call me and I'll be on my way, okay? Otherwise, I'll see you on June . . ."

"Twenty-first, at 10 A.M.," she finished.

"Right," I snapped back eagerly. "But don't forget what I said about the waiting list, okay?"

"Two hours away, a full tank of gas," she repeated.

Being a stand-by patient was better than nothing; I honestly didn't believe I could hang on until June. Physically, I was in bad shape. Every symptom I'd ever had was present nearly every day. I was always exhausted, and sometimes didn't make it to work until almost noon. My mind fog was so bad I couldn't make sense out of the Sunday paper. But there was something else compelling me to push for that appointment, something beyond the pain and confusion. I needed a name for what all of this was. I needed some sort of vindication. I needed someone in the medical profession to come through for me, to take what I had to say seriously, to not just ask if I were simply under a lot of stress.

On Thursday, March 1, Dr. Cheney's receptionist called. There had been a last-minute cancellation. I'd get my March 2 appointment after all.

8

APPOINTMENT IN CHARLOTTE

Hettie and I hurriedly left Florence that evening and drove to Charlotte. It was a mild night, and as soon as we got there, we stopped at a phone booth and Hettie called for a hotel room. My brain fog was so thick that I wasn't able to read the telephone book or take directions. I remember shaking violently, as if I were stuck inside a deep-freeze. I'd been so wrapped up in my efforts to make this appointment happen that I'd slipped back into feeling immortal, but this uncontrollable shaking changed that. Something *had* to be wrong with me. The rest of the way to the hotel I rode in silence, pondering the reality that this trip was more a result of my failing health than my ability to come up with a good plan.

The next morning at exactly 10 A.M., Hettie and I arrived at Dr. Cheney's. I brought all my test results from my other doctors' visits and the emergency room trips, and Hettie was prepared to take notes. *The Hunt for Red October*, the long-awaited film version of Tom Clancy's novel, was to debut that night in theaters across the country. We stopped along the way to buy a *USA Today* to read about the movie. In the few minutes we spent in Dr. Cheney's small waiting room, I tried to read the page-one story about the movie. My mind was so jumbled that I couldn't figure out where on the page to start! I dropped the paper, feeling a breeze of fear blow across my body. I prayed that I was in the right place.

After completing some paperwork, Hettie and I settled into an exam room to await the arrival of the Wizard. From past experience, I figured we'd be waiting until almost lunchtime, but fifteen minutes later the tall, sandy-haired doctor I had read about just two weeks earlier strode into the room. The brief time I spent waiting for Dr. Cheney was more than the entire time I had actually spent with every doctor I had seen for the past two years.

"I'm Paul Cheney," he said softly, and shook my hand. He apologized for making us wait. "Seeing patients and doing research is a hard thing to do," he explained, "but it's very necessary. I got tied up on the phone." He apologized again.

I could tell I was dealing with a doctor very different from any I had ever met. The "you-wait-for-me" arrogance just wasn't a part of this guy's style. I relaxed a bit, and Cheney began his physical exam, which was not a whole lot different from the exams I had to get for my pilot's license. I remember that he felt my lymph nodes carefully and palpated my spleen. In both cases, I winced in pain.

After he checked my reflexes in places I didn't know I had any, he asked me to stand on one foot at a time, then with feet front-to-back and my arms extended.

While I was in the latter position, he made an unusual request. "Subtract seven from one hundred."

"Ninety-three," I hastily answered. I was losing my balance.

"Seven from ninety-three?" he asked.

I paused, stunned. I had always been first in my class to complete tests, doing calculations in my head even when the teacher insisted on seeing the work. I was a commercial-rated pilot who had nearly aced three FAA tests in record time. Now I couldn't even do a simple math problem. *Ninety-three minus seven*. I guessed at the answer and missed. Cheney asked me to subtract seven a few more times, and I just kept guessing.

After concluding the exam, Cheney invited us to follow him into his office. There, he explained what the CDC had settled upon as diagnostic criteria for CFS. He had a checklist in front of him, and from my questionnaire, other medical records, and his exam notes, he began checking off the boxes. In a few moments, he placed his pen in front of him, looked up at me, and spoke quite softly. "You do meet the published criteria for this syndrome."

He continued, telling us that he would order some additional blood tests to rule out Lyme disease and a few other disorders, and to study various markers in my immune system. But for me, there in black and white on his desk was the answer I had been yearning for. I was a textbook case of this thing called chronic fatigue syndrome.

I find it hard to describe my feelings at that moment. Oddly, I recall a sense of relief. Technically, I didn't know a thing about this disease, although my body had been telling me about it for months. At least now I knew its name. Now I could find a way to take it on, a way to win. I had to fight to hold back tears of relief. I thought I knew what I was up against—*finally!* The process could be a breeze from here, I reasoned optimistically.

This very temporary sense of relief is nearly universal among CFS patients when they finally get a diagnosis. In most cases, after years of fighting a medical establishment that refuses to accept the illness, it is indeed a relief to meet a doctor who finally agrees that something is wrong. That's all we initially want: a diagnosis, a starting point, something to fight.

After leaving Dr. Cheney, I went to a nearby laboratory and had several tubes of blood drawn for the tests. I was scheduled for a six-week follow-up with Cheney's assistant to review the lab work. I would see the Wizard himself again in early July, but the PA would discuss some preliminary test results. I also left Cheney's office with a fistful of prescriptions to help combat the exhaustion, neurological problems, and sleeplessness that was plaguing me. More important than the medicine, though, I left with the hope that finally someone would be trying to help me get well.

Hettie and I were quiet in the car driving back to our hotel. We weren't sure if we'd gotten good news or bad news, but I think we both sensed we were about to take on something bigger than we'd ever fought before. We decided to stay over another night in Charlotte and after an afternoon nap, we went to see *Red October*. Submarine movies are among my favorites, and I think we both just needed some time to take in all that Dr. Cheney had said during our three-hour visit. The movie was a timely distraction.

The relief I felt in Dr. Cheney's office turned out to be very short-lived. My symptoms all continued, and many of them even worsened. Knowing the name of my illness did not make it go away.

9

GOING COLD TURKEY

The first stop Hettie and I made when we returned to our hometown was at a small pharmacy. Since we had several prescriptions to be filled and suspected that we'd be getting a lot more filled on a regular basis, we wanted to find an understanding pharmacist with whom we could build a relationship.

Among the prescriptions Dr. Cheney had given me was one for a tricyclic antidepressant. Usually such medication is tried soon after a CFS diagnosis is given, but not to combat depression. As volumes of research have proved, CFS is not depression, is not related to depression, and its clinical markers have nothing in common with those of depression. Instead, the antidepressants may be prescribed to help regulate a substance in the brain called serotonin. But the dosage prescribed for this purpose is often a tiny fraction—perhaps ten percent—of what might be prescribed for depression. A prescription for such a low dosage of a fairly common family of medicines might seem a bit unusual to the average pharmacist, who knows nothing about CFS.

"We don't stock it like this," the pharmacist behind the counter sniffed.

"Can you get it?" I asked.

"Why would you want it like this?" he asked, almost antagonistic.

Now a year's worth of medical frustration was surfacing in me. "Because that's how my doctor ordered it," I said curtly. "If you don't have it, who would?"

"This late on a Saturday afternoon? You've got no chance of finding this concoction anywhere in town."

This guy was really getting on what was left of my frayed nerves. I hated the idea of giving him one penny's worth of my business, but I was sick and tired of running around looking for answers. I decided I'd done without the drugs for this long, so another few days wouldn't hurt.

"Fine," I said sternly. "Order it."

He looked up at me, mystified. He had the stronger version of the stuff right there, and I could have it right then and get on with getting over my depression.

Well, I wasn't depressed, and I wasn't in the mood to negotiate any longer. I wanted the drugs that Dr. Cheney had ordered exactly as he had ordered them, and I wanted them yesterday. I succeeded in communicating that point to the man behind the counter, and I went home and climbed into bed.

After a few more such encounters and several strange looks from this pharmacist, we took our business to a small, family-owned drugstore near Hettie's office. The people at Dixon Drug became instant friends. They took an interest in me and my case, even researching CFS and sending me copies of several magazine articles on the subject. They became very close with Hettie and exchanged Christmas presents and other pleasantries as time passed, and whenever I would stop in, they'd always treat me with courtesy and respect. On the day we moved away from Florence, I stopped in to say goodbye to those great people, and they invited me to pick out my own going-away present from their selection of jigsaw puzzles. And months after we were no longer customers, they remembered us at Christmas, as well.

My experience with pharmacies proved, as my experience with physicians did, that you don't have to put up with abuse as a patient. You may have to keep looking, but there are decent, kind, competent people willing to help.

The annoying pharmacist was not the only one giving me strange looks or making unfeeling comments. Less than a week after I returned from Charlotte, one of my employees stopped by my office after returning from an appointment with her gynecologist.

"I told my doctor about what your doctor said," she announced.

I didn't look up from the news story I was editing. I really didn't care what any other doctors said, but my obvious disinterest didn't deter my colleague from sharing the medical misinformation her doctor had passed on.

"*He* says the only people who get chronic fatigue syndrome are people who have two thousand dollars to spend on blood tests." She seemed almost breathless with excitement in sharing this revelation.

Her comment stung me, badly. I threw down my pen and nearly leapt across the desk. I cursed out loud and demanded the name of this doctor who, with neither apparent expertise in CFS nor knowledge of me, felt he could sum up my case so glibly. The notion that someone thought I had "bought" my diagnosis infuriated me, and I wanted to let him know that.

My colleague balked for a moment, but when I continued to express my anger—now in her direction—she finally muttered the doctor's name. Then she hastily retreated from my office, mumbling that she only thought I should consider getting a second opinion.

I knew what both she and her doctor meant; they didn't believe CFS existed. Like so many uninformed physicians who do not understand emerging disorders, this doctor assumed that since CFS was outside the realm of his knowledge, it could not be a real disease. I wondered how many patients had wasted their precious time, money, and energy on the likes of this man. And since a majority of CFS patients are women, that number must have been pretty high. (We are just beginning to notice the discrimination against female patients by the medical profession.)

I immediately wrote a strongly worded letter to the offending doctor, telling him what I knew about CFS and urging him to find out more before making such a callous comment again, especially to one of his own—perhaps very ill—patients. I sent him more information in the coming year, including a government pamphlet for physicians as soon as it was published. He never wrote back. I still remember this doctor's name, and I hope he and I don't meet on a dark street some night when I am strong and healthy again. To me, he represents all the doctors who didn't take me seriously; and all the doctors who have dismissed women's complaints as depression, moodiness, or PMS. As with the uncooperative pharmacist, I had plenty of anger to share with this physician. I can tolerate doubt—especially in a profession that requires some skepticism—but I have no patience for outright hostility and abuse and the physicians who dole it out without thinking. I recall this man often, and I speak of him and his ignorance whenever I talk with a newly diagnosed CFS patient. No matter where they live, no matter what doctors they have seen, virtually every patient I have met has come across this man or his ilk.

My own road to diagnosis was a relatively short one, but I know of one patient who went to more than two hundred doctors before being diagnosed with CFS. Another sufferer who is a leader in the CFS patient network was actually sent to a mental ward before finally being diagnosed correctly.

Fortunately, some people were sympathetic and open about my condition. My boss was supportive after hearing my account of the Cheney visit, and I'll always be grateful for that. The president of our company suffered from multiple sclerosis, so all of our company's station managers were sensitive to illness. Unfortunately, I cannot say the same about all of my co-workers.

Within a few weeks, word that "Tim is faking it" began to be spread by some people who apparently didn't have anything better to do with their time. Apparently unable to believe that something was physically wrong with me, or perhaps looking for any opportunity to advance themselves at another's expense, they forced me to lose time and energy looking over my shoulder. It seems senseless to have to defend oneself against that sort of petty thinking, but it's a necessary self-preservation measure in the back-biting business world.

The medications Dr. Cheney had ordered seemed to help my sleeplessness a bit, but they did little else for my other symptoms. I still felt like a mere shell of a person—sapped of all energy and struggling just to make it through each day. Some nights after work I was so wracked with pain that Hettie had to help me from the car. The days that went by with only minor discomfort were becoming much less frequent.

On April 17, Dr. Cheney ordered a more specific test for Lyme disease. The first test had been inconclusive, but this one came back definitely negative. On April 26, about seven weeks after my first meeting with Cheney, I met with his PA to go over my lab results. In preparation, I had glanced through a couple of books about the immune system, and so I at least was somewhat familiar with the terminology.

Despite my new knowledge, what I learned in that meeting astounded me. Many components of my immune system were running at full throttle, and some of them were now actually toxic to my brain and body. This was the case with nearly all CFS patients.

How could a system that's supposed to protect the body attack it this way? Consider what happens when you get the flu. When you first get it, you feel next to death—no one in history has ever felt this sick. But its not the influenza virus itself that makes you feel so lousy. For the most part, it's your body's own immune response, including chemicals called cytokines, that makes you feel so awful. That's why CFS patients feel so terrible—they have a wide-open immune system.

The level of alpha-interferon (a chemical produced by the immune system in response to viruses and other invaders) in my blood was enough to be toxic, the PA told me. In fact, it was the highest they'd seen to date. Other immunological markers were similarly skewed. My immune system was either fighting an invisible invader, or was being fooled into fighting an invader that wasn't there. In either case, *I* was the main casualty. That's why I was feeling so awful all the time. I really did have a flu that just wouldn't quit.

Paradoxically, those initial tests also revealed that some components of my immune system were virtually shut down. This seeming contradiction suggested that if a virus had invaded my body, it was playing multiple tricks on my immune system or even damaging various parts of it. It turns out that what we refer to as "the immune system" is really dozens of separate systems. Some of my systems were going a hundred miles an hour, while others were idling.

The PA also told me of some doctors in Texas who'd achieved excellent results with CFS patients using an antiinflammatory drug called Kutapressin. After looking at their data, I was immediately impressed and asked to try the treatment. For the next several months, I injected myself with the drug more than a hundred and fifty times, with no noticeable results except the needle marks on my arms. I was happy for the people who'd been helped by Kutapressin, but it clearly wasn't a solution for me. Like the small-dose antidepressants, Kutapressin became one of the many hopes that turned into disappointments in my treatment protocol.

The annual Sun Fun Festival came around again in June 1990, three months after my CFS diagnosis. The people at *Good Morning America* declined my offer to come back for a third appearance, which was fortunate for me. By that time, I had learned the art of delegating responsibility, and I just survived the week. By Sunday night I could barely walk.

On Tuesday, July 10, I had another appointment with Dr. Cheney. I had been trying to learn all I could about T-cells, CD4 cells, natural killer cells, helper cells, suppressor cells, and all the other immune cells so that I could follow along with Cheney's explanations. If I was going to have a hand in fighting this disease, I had to know all I could about it. But the subject is so complex that, in a matter of minutes after the appointment began, Dr. Cheney was discussing some aspect of my blood work that was way beyond anything I had learned.

"It's this cellular ratio right here that concerns me," he said, circling some lab results he had already marked.

I looked at him, awaiting an explanation.

"We have seen it in a few CFS patients," he went on, "but it's quite a bit more common in another disease."

"What disease?" I asked. I'd already had extra tests to rule out autoimmune disorders and connective tissue diseases and cancers and tumors and dozens of other things I'd never heard of before. I expected Dr. Cheney to name some bizarre, unknown disorder that would send me again to the medical encyclopedias.

"AIDS," he said softly. "I want to test you for HIV."

I didn't fit any of the publicized AIDS risk groups and was a regular blood donor until I had gotten sick, so I'd never given any thought to AIDS. Now the one doctor I trusted was telling me it was a possibility. I had heard CFS compared to a life sentence. AIDS was more like a death sentence.

Using a specially coded tube, an assistant drew some blood from my right arm, and Dr. Cheney changed the subject, dismissing the HIV test as little more than a formality.

I asked about Ampligen, an experimental drug, that I'd heard about. It had been tested on only a dozen or so CFS patients, with mixed but encouraging results. That sounded positive to me, and since nothing else had worked, I wanted to try anything.

Cheney passed me to one of his nurses who explained the coming Ampligen trial, part of the long and involved process that drug companies go through to get FDA approval for their products. In all such efforts, human trials are needed, and often the sickest people are chosen because they have little to lose if the drug doesn't work. The nurse told me that there would be many tests, some of them painful, and reams of paperwork before I was accepted for the trial. And I would have to immediately go cold turkey off all my other medications, even aspirin.

The medications weren't giving me much relief anyway, except allowing me to catch a few hours of sleep each night. My health was deteriorating rapidly, and I felt as if I was running out of options. Though Ampligen was essentially untried, it sounded like a chance for me to regain my life. I measured the risks against the potential benefits, and knew what I had to do.

"Sign me up," I said.

That simple statement began one of the most intense and emotional periods in my life. In the next two years, I'd see my health nearly restored for a brief time and then slip away, I'd threaten a major lawsuit against the drug's manufacturer, and I'd be stuck with hundreds of IV needles.

* * *

Driving home from Charlotte that afternoon, I focused again on the AIDS test. Like most Americans in 1990, I was sadly uninformed about the disease. I did know that it left no survivors. I looked at the bandage on my arm, and I wanted to rip it off as if doing so would make the horror of what I was thinking about go away. I wanted to take my blood back, to tear up the consent form for the test, to stop the whole rotten process.

In the next few days, I learned what it is like to face the possibility of being infected with the AIDS virus. The waiting is terrible.

I decided not to call Cheney's office for the test results. Each time I had gone through another test ordered by Dr. Cheney in the past months, it seemed as if the news was always bad. Some new thing was always way out of line; some new problem was always turning up. It was denial that kept me from making the call. If I ignored the possibility that I could have AIDS, I reasoned, I wouldn't—I *couldn't*—have AIDS.

Finally, Cheney's office called me. I had stopped by my house for a moment one afternoon and was about to leave when the phone rang. I rushed into the bedroom to grab it before the answering machine picked up.

"May I speak to Tim Kenny, please?" the polite female voice asked. I could tell it was Sheryl Autry, a nurse in Dr. Cheney's office.

"This is Tim Kenny," I said, a chill passing through my body. My knees buckled, and I sank onto the edge of the bed. The telephone receiver slipped in my hand as I broke out in a cold sweat.

"Mr. Kenny, this is Sheryl from Dr. Cheney's office, and I'm calling about . . ."

"Yes, I know," I interrupted. Everything else had turned out poorly. All of the other tests had turned up something bad. This one did, too—I was sure. I knew what she was going to tell me, and I held my breath.

"Everything is just fine. The test was negative."

I blinked, and then let out a long breath. I didn't have AIDS.

I placed the receiver back on the nightstand with trembling hands. I laid on the bed for a long time before I was composed enough to move.

My involvement with FDA-approved protocol #502, the first double-blind multi-site Ampligen trial, began in July 1990 with those early questions to Dr. Cheney and his staff. In the weeks and months after that, my entire life—and my health—would center on Ampligen as they had on no other influence before. I really had no idea what I was getting myself into, and I don't know whether I would ever do it again. Ampligen certainly changed my life in many ways, some for the better, some for the worse. Its short-term effect on my health was dramatic; its long-term impact won't be known for years.

Shortly after I learned of the coming trial, I pursued being included in the study with all of the vigor and determination I could muster. First I wrote an emphatic letter to Janie Warlick, the nurse in Dr. Cheney's office who would be supervising the study there. I made my case in demonstrative terms; I wanted to be a part of the experiment, and I would do anything to make that happen.

With Janie's help, I soon embarked on the long, tortuous path that would lead me to what I hoped would be my miracle cure. The first thing I had to do was discontinue all of my medications. These included Klonopin for neurological symptoms, Sinequon and Prozac to stimulate the immune system, something for sleep, injecting Toridol for pain twice a day, injecting Kutapressin, an antiinflammatory, Lioresol for muscle spasticity, among others. The withdrawal was terrifying. Night after night I would toss about in bed, unable to grab even an hour's rest. I spent many days at work with my head exploding in pain. And I experienced terrible new symptoms from the withdrawal on top of what the CFS was doing to me.

Acting on the information she'd been given, Janie had told me that my first Ampligen infusion would probably come in about six weeks, meaning that I would start on the experimental protocol in late August or early September. There was much to be done in that period, including verifying one more time that I did indeed have CFS.

CFS was and still is very much a diagnosis of exclusion; that is, once a patient *appears* to have the syndrome, all other possible explanations must be eliminated. That's why I had had the AIDS test. There was no specific test for CFS then, and still none today. Thus, as I stood in line to be considered for the Ampligen experiment, I underwent dozens of expensive and sometimes painful tests to rule out all other maladies.

I had another MRI scan of my brain to check for possible tumors and lesions. I suffered through a lumbar puncture—the worst procedure I have ever been through—to rule out multiple sclerosis and other disorders. I had countless blood tests aimed at eliminating all manner of strange ailments. I even had at least one pregnancy test.

A lot of initial paperwork had to be tackled, as well. A detailed medical history had to be constructed, I had to produce all previous medical records, and I had to fill out a number of screening questionnaires, presumably to prove that I was not suffering from any psychiatric disorders. My baseline IQ values were determined by specialists flown in from the University of California at Berkeley. (One of the strangest symptoms of advanced CFS cases is a decrease in IQ; my own values had dropped nearly forty points). I endured two exhausting treadmill tests to measure baseline cardiovascular function and how efficiently my body used oxygen and produced carbon dioxide.

I began to keep track of my own abilities using a form called an Assessment of Daily Living (ADL). The initial ADLs would also be used as baselines for comparison throughout the study. In addition, specially coded blood samples were sent to laboratories all over the country where scientists would study various markers in my immune system before, during, and after the Ampligen trial.

I endured all of this knowing that I had only a fifty percent chance of actually receiving Ampligen. The trial was to be a double-blind test, so neither clinicians nor patients would know who was getting the drug and who was getting a placebo. As the weeks went by, the tests piled up and the emotional drain increased.

One day I vented the strain to Bill Christian. "I just don't know if all this trouble is worth a fifty-fifty chance of getting Ampligen," I told him. Early in the testing period, I had told Bill that I would put up with almost anything because HEM Pharmaceuticals, the manufacturer, had promised that the placebo recipients would be transferred to Ampligen once the study was concluded and the Ampligen recipients would continue on the drug indefinitely.

Bill was the voice of reason that I needed to hear to keep me going. "What choice do you have? Aren't there something like *millions* of people with this disease, and aren't there only going to be one hundred and twenty on the study? It seems to me that you need to do anything you can to at least hold your place in line for the Ampligen."

Once again, my resolve to be included in the study was restored.

As summer waned, I kept calling Nurse Warlick to ask when I would start my infusions. All she could do was tell me the latest word from HEM Pharmaceuticals. Week after agonizing week— Labor Day passed, then Columbus Day, then Halloween—I endured the delay. My symptoms were back with a vengeance, and my overall health was continuing its steady decline.

Through it all, Janie Warlick was fantastic. I have never met an individual placed in such an undesirable position who conducted herself so admirably. On the one hand, she had a horde of impatient patients like me who wanted the trial to start yesterday. On the other hand, she had HEM Pharmaceuticals, which seemed to be taking an answer-of-the-week attitude toward requests for information about the trial. I don't know what kept Janie going through all of that, what helped her maintain her professional, caring demeanor, stuck as she was between a rock and a hard place. I can only presume that Janie possesses a sum total of goodness sufficient to outweigh all the abuses and ignorance I had encountered in medicine before I ever met her.

* * *

Three important events unrelated to preparing for the Ampligen trial took place around this time. First, in mid-June I attended a meeting of the Charlotte-area CFIDS support group. (Though I use CFS—the government's poorly chosen name for the disease— in this book, many clinicians and patients have adopted CFIDS— chronic fatigue and immune dysfunction syndrome, a much more accurate name.) The featured speaker that night was Dr. Tarras Onischenko, a Brazilian-born Ph.D. practicing in the Charlotte area. Dr. Onischenko specializes in neuropsychology and cognitive rehabilitation. He was speaking on things like memory problems and mind fog when the topic of head injuries came up.

"I think that any kind of trauma to the brain predisposes the brain to further problems in the future," Onischenko responded to a question. (His remarks were later reprinted in *The CFIDS Chronicle*, the journal published by the CFIDS Association.) "I really do believe that. So, if you've had a head injury, let's say ten years ago, I think your brain, although it may be intact and functional, isn't the brain it was ten years ago and that if there is encephalopathy [a viral infection], I think it's more likely to be predisposed. So I think the brain is more compromised and more susceptible to other problems."

I thought of my concussion. This explained why my neurological and cognitive symptoms were so profound. Normally, the blood-brain barrier keeps all but the most severe infections (and most medications) from reaching the brain. Coming just after that bug bite in the Bahamas, which I suspected was my initial infection, the concussion opened my brain up for a direct attack.

I didn't feel any better about my illness that night, but Dr. Onischenko's explanation helped me understand it.

The second significant event occurred on July 11, the first day I went cold turkey from my medications. I was driving a brand-new Chevrolet S-10 that had just been detailed with our station's logo, and I smashed it into another car. The S-10 was almost totally wrecked, but I was able to call the station for help on the two-way radio.

"What happened?" my producer asked when he arrived a few minutes later.

I didn't know, and I still don't know. My mind had simply jumbled things up for a moment. I sat in that wrecked truck for the longest time with my head in my hands. I wasn't upset about some bent-up sheet metal and plastic. I was just wondering what was happening with my life.

The third event, which I deeply regret, happened on September 21. I'd been off all medications for more than two months, I hadn't had a decent night's sleep in that time, and I was almost always in a state of agitation. The Ampligen trial, which was supposed to start in six weeks, had been delayed, and I couldn't get straight information on when it would begin. And I had been working for weeks on a number of special TV projects surrounding the one-year anniversary of Hurricane Hugo.

One of those projects was something entirely of my doing, an event called a satellite media tour. The idea was to show a completely healed and restored Myrtle Beach to the rest of the country, since the last TV images of the area had been of the destruction immediately following Hugo. The local business community had turned to our station for help, I proposed the satellite media tour, and the project landed in my lap.

We brought a satellite truck and a producer in from New York, and booked local author Mickey Spillane in newscasts and on talk-shows all over the country. Spillane—creator of the Mike Hammer character in books, movies, and a television show—lived just south of Myrtle Beach, and we'd been acquainted since my days as a radio reporter. I figured his notoriety, plus the fact that he'd lost his home to Hugo, would make him an instant attraction as an interview subject. Wearing his omnipresent Lite Beer shirt, Spillane would be interviewed live from the beautifully manicured beach by TV news anchors and talk-show hosts in markets from New York to Nashville to Phoenix. Spillane would also get the chance to plug his beer sponsor as well as his latest book, written to finance the rebuilding of his home.

I'd personally done a similar interview that day for a station in

Pittsburgh, since I was originally from the Pittsburgh area and had done some part-time work for the station a decade earlier. I tried to arrange other such appearances for some of my staff, giving them the chance to appear as hurricane survivors on stations in their hometowns. I even tried to set up a hometown appearance for one guy from a competing station whose home was in Cincinnati.

Tom Dewees and I were casual friends. I really wanted to get Tom on TV where his parents would see him and be proud. Despite my efforts, the producers in Cincinnati opted for neither Tom nor Mickey Spillane, but for my news anchor. Tom and I were both disappointed and a bit confused by the choice, but I was too busy coordinating the daylong event to discuss it with him. When I finally arrived home that night, I heard from a co-worker that Tom was saying that I had intentionally passed him over to get someone else on TV, costing him his only chance to be on the air back home.

I exploded when I heard the story. The notion of being so mis-understood and unappreciated boiled up inside of me. For some reason, I went out looking for Tom, feeling like I wanted to kill him. My brain must have been a real wreck, because I was like a man possessed, virtually out of control. I found Tom in a restaurant only a mile from my home, and I dragged him outside. I screamed at him, demanding an explanation.

Tom quickly apologized, and that calmed me down. My irra-tional rage drained slowly, and reason returned. But looking back on the incident, I know I was out of control and could easily have hurt this decent man. To this day when I see Tom, I apologize pro-fusely, often having to dab away tears of shame for what I did. He's a fine fellow, a friend and former colleague, and I nearly ripped his head off. I know it wasn't the real me who attacked Tom that way; that my illness and the drug withdrawal made me do it; but the thought of that evening still makes me shudder in fear.

10

THE AMPLIGEN TRIAL

It was Thanksgiving week, and the moment had finally arrived. My miracle cure hung on a pole just eighteen inches above my head. From the glass bottle, a tube snaked through an IV pump, dropped over my shoulder, and then followed down my arm to a needle inserted into a vein on the top of my hand, deftly slid into place just a moment earlier by Sheryl Autry.

Sheryl programmed the IV pump by pressing some buttons, and then smiled at me. "All ready?" she asked.

Ready? I'd been ready for this since Dr. Cheney told me about the Ampligen trial in July. I'd been writing letters, making phone calls, submitting to dozens of tests, and doing anything else I could to become a part of the Ampligen trial. And even though I knew there was only a fifty-fifty chance that the bottle above my head actually contained the real drug and not a placebo, I was already imagining its healing powers.

I glanced over to my brother Bob, who had come with me for this first infusion. Then I nodded to Sheryl, and she pressed the start button. The fluid began coming down the tube and into my hand. Sheryl checked the area around the needle and, satisfied that all was well, slid an emergency call button in front of Betty, another trial participant who was receiving her dose at the same time, and stepped out of the room.

And then it happened.

At first, I felt as if a pair of hands were around my neck, choking off my breathing. I struggled for air, and tried to blink back the tears that were now pouring from my eyes. Suddenly, my skin felt as if it were on fire, and a terrible itching enveloped me.

"Tim, are you all right?" Betty asked.

I nodded that I was, but my appearance belied my assurance. My eyes were wide with fear and I was turning beet-red. Bob, a paramedic, was watching me closely, and must have immediately recognized the signs of an allergic reaction.

"Can you breathe?" he asked.

"I'm okay," I croaked. "Just give me a minute."

"Want me to call Sheryl?" Betty asked, reaching for the call button.

With my free hand, I signaled her to leave the button alone. After all I had done to beat the odds just to get into this trial, I was either going to get well or die trying.

Bob was measuring my racing pulse and watching me for a cue as to what he should do. I was allergic to one other drug— Tylenol—and I hoped that this reaction would soon subside just as my reactions to Tylenol had. But this was an experimental drug, and I was a test case. Would I become one of those "rare fatal reactions" that I'd read about on prescription inserts?

Three or four minutes passed, and the reaction did not diminish. The thought crossed my mind that I was heading for anaphylactic shock, that my heart could seize up and my breathing stop, that I could die. But I was determined to endure the choking, the horrible itch, and the burning sensation for as long as I possibly could. I prayed that Sheryl wouldn't come back into the room and spot my condition, which would end my involvement in the Ampligen trial the very hour it had begun.

Finally the reaction began to subside. By the time Sheryl did return, I was still red-faced and teary-eyed, but I was breathing more normally and my heart had slowed its frantic pace.

"Are you feeling okay?" she asked, slowing the IV drip.

"Umm, fine," I said, clearing my throat. "Just a little reaction, but it's almost gone."

From that moment on, Sheryl and I had our own special code. When I said I was "fine," it meant that I was really feeling absolutely terrible. It also meant I didn't want any help, I didn't want to quit. Even now when she asks me how I'm doing and I answer "fine," she knows it's my way of saying I'm doing awful, but there's nothing we can do about it.

Sheryl turned to my brother and asked his opinion.

"I think he'll be okay in a second," Bob said.

I never was really "okay" during the infusion, but I survived it. A half hour later I breathed a sigh of relief as Sheryl slipped the needle out of my hand.

In that half hour, I went from being Tim Kenny to being Ampligen patient 059. Although the trial was a double-blind study in which neither clinicians nor patients knew who was getting drug and who was getting placebo, I was certain that the bottles I received twice each week contained the real McCoy. You simply don't have that kind of a reaction to saline.

Now that I knew I was getting it, the real test would be whether I would have some sort of positive response to Ampligen.

The earliest Greek playwrights used a rhetorical device called *deus ex machina* to get their characters out of seemingly inescapable messes. Literally translated, the expression means "God as machine," but it refers to an instant solution, or an unexpected and divine answer to a host of overwhelming problems. Centuries later, television sitcom writers would revive this technique, managing to create and solve a host of problems for their characters in twenty-two minutes. Looking back at that first Ampligen infusion, I think I was expecting the same type of tidy fix for my own terrible situation. Unfortunately, what worked in those early Greek plays and in today's mindless sitcoms did not work in real life—or in *my* real life, in any case. The quick fix never came.

In fact, in December 1990 and on into January 1991, my health actually seemed to get worse from being on the Ampligen. This was the initial "crash," and it seemed pretty universal among the patients who were receiving the drug. And the stress of the grueling twice-weekly trips to Charlotte, which I had ignored in my eagerness to be part of the study, were taking their own serious toll on me.

For the first few months of the study, I left home before sunrise for the two-hour-plus drive to Charlotte. I'd arrive at Dr. Cheney's office at 8:15 A.M., leave by 9:00, and be back in my office a little before 11:00. Sometimes I'd even beat one of the other department heads to the television station, despite my five-hour commute.

But as my health worsened, it became harder for me to face the early morning drive to Charlotte. And often, for an hour or so after the infusion, I was sluggish and had a rough time staying on the road. I knew I had to either change my schedule or quit the Ampligen study. In the back of my mind lurked a third option—move to Charlotte—but that seemed out of the question. I had a career and a life in South Carolina. Admittedly, both were in decline, but I was hoping that the Ampligen would change all of that.

At about the time that Operation Desert Storm began and U.S. bombers started to bomb Iraq, in the middle of January, I finally decided to change my schedule for the infusions. Units from the nearby Myrtle Beach Air Force Base had been deployed to the Gulf, and they were playing a major role in the air campaign against Iraq. In addition, several local National Guard and Reserve groups were taking part in the war as well. Our television station was as involved in the coverage as any local station in America, and the demands on my time were incredible. And I had sent two of my own people to Saudi Arabia to report on our local troops. I felt personally responsible for them, and knew I needed to be back in the office early every morning to assess the situation. So I decided I would come to work first, plan our coverage for the day and supervise the goings-on for a while, and then head to Charlotte around noon. I would get to Dr. Cheney's a little after two o'clock and still get back to the station before the six o'clock news.

Despite my illness and the demands of the Ampligen trial, I remained an active news director. Always the investigative reporter, I had obtained some secret telephone numbers for an air base in the Gulf, and would call for a daily report on our local troops' well-being. A stern phone call from a government agency threatening to charge me with a breach of national security put a stop to that. But I was always on the phone with my reporters, whether they were down the block or on the other side of the world. As I drove to Charlotte, I had my cellular phone constantly to my ear, always making plans or decisions, always consulting with my producer or my general manager, always trying to keep up the appearance of being fully functional. My ultimate goal remained producing the best newscast possible—the pledge that had gotten me the job in the first place. Thousands of families in our viewing area had someone in the Gulf, and I felt a responsibility to them all. My mobile phone bills climbed to several hundred dollars a month during this period, but I considered it simply another cost of my illness.

The new schedule seemed to be a little easier on me. By the time Operation Desert Storm was over in early March, I was feeling better than I had for over a year. The Ampligen appeared to be helping. I looked forward to continuing to receive the drug and continuing to improve.

As I neared my sixth month on the drug study, the Charlotte Ampligen patients were summoned to a special meeting early one evening. Dr. Cheney's nurses and even a patient counselor were on hand. We all sensed the serious mood of the meeting, even before the announcement was made: HEM Pharmaceuticals would end the drug trial at six months—not a year—and the company was breaking its promise that we would receive Ampligen afterward. HEM had enough data to apply for drug approval, and they no longer had need to continue the expensive experimental protocol. We were about to be cast aside like used test tubes.

I left the meeting early, choosing not to engage in the angry discussion that followed the announcement. We were all understandably furious, but I knew there was nothing to be gained by blowing off steam there; I had a long drive home and much to consider.

Perhaps to appease the study group, HEM initially announced that any patient deemed a "significant responder" to Ampligen would be kept on the drug, even after the early end of the study. But HEM never announced its criteria for determining who fit the category, and those of us involved in the study felt this was just a feeble attempt to show some sensitivity toward us. As for the rest of the promises HEM had made when we'd agreed to be in the study, the company simply had nothing to say. There would be no switch to Ampligen for the placebo patients and no open-label continuation for the Ampligen patients.

By mid-May, with just two weeks remaining in my six-month period, I was consumed with the reality of what was about to happen. I was feeling and functioning better than I had at any time since I'd become ill, and I was about to be yanked off the drug that I believed had made this all possible. I'd sacrificed in untold ways to be in the study; I'd made severe financial and career compromises, my waning social life had completely collapsed, and I had allowed my body to become a laboratory for an experimental concoction that nearly killed me the first time I received it. I had done all of this for the promise of receiving Ampligen until its ultimate approval by the FDA, and now that promise was being yanked away.

Study patients around the country began to revolt in their own ways. Many wrote letters, called government agencies, visited congresspeople, circulated petitions, and whatever else they knew to do. Some began to talk about hiring attorneys. Others talked of a deepening depression caused by the broken promise of a brighter future.

I concentrated on finding out what HEM meant by the term "significant responder." No one seemed to be able to tell me. Was the response it was looking for in our treadmill tests, our IQ assessment, our daily living logs, or somewhere deep in the hidden recesses of all the blood tests it was conducting? Or was it looking for the recommendation of the doctors and nurses who'd administered the trial? Despite my best investigative efforts, I couldn't find out, and I grew angry and anxious as my cut-off day neared.

I knew that my final battery of tests would show that I'd improved dramatically since starting on Ampligen, and I reasoned that such a response should move me into the "responder" category. But since I didn't know HEM's criteria—or even if criteria actually existed—I began to consider proving on my own that I had responded to Ampligen.

I went to a trusted friend and attorney, the same man who had represented me and the station in several lawsuits. It's not unusual to be sued when you're in the television news business, and it had happened to me three times. Each time this attorney and I had won. In this upcoming battle, I told him, we might actually be fighting for my life.

Our strategy would be simple: Ampligen had made a difference in my life, and it would be unethical for HEM to deny me access to the drug that was helping me so much. I used the analogy of a drowning swimmer—how cruel it would be to throw someone a lifeline and then cut it as he were nearing safety. We would argue that Ampligen had rescued me from drowning in CFS. The drug company had originally promised to continue Ampligen for all of us; we felt it had a compelling reason to keep its promise, especially for those of us who had responded to the experimental treatment.

Once again, I discovered how lucky I was to have an enlightened employer. I had no idea how I would pay the attorney's fees and court costs of my proposed action, since my travel and other expenses related to my illness were eating into my salary. Diversified Communications, the company that owned WPDE, held a conference call with Bill Christian to discuss how they could help. When I think of the hundreds of thousands of CFS patients whose employers treat them unfairly because of this misunderstood and poorly named illness, I give thanks that I was working for such a compassionate company. The people at Diversified might not have known much about CFS, but they were convinced of two things: I was sick, and I needed help.

Bill called me into his office after the call. "You know there's nothing we can do to help you under the health insurance plan," Bill began. I nodded, having earlier pored over the company policy book and questioned our benefits administrator a day or so earlier.

"But there is something we can do that doesn't have anything to do with insurance," Bill continued. "It's not nearly enough, but we just want to help you get started. Your legal fees will probably be ten times this much, but we want you to have this just to know we care."

With that, he handed me a check for one thousand dollars. Bill called it a "performance bonus," and tried to assure me that my job performance had been superb despite my health problems. I knew I'd been working hard when others would have given up, but I took the check for what it was—a gift.

I didn't know what to say. Our company didn't typically give bonuses, at least not to sick news directors. I asked Bill how we could afford it given the tight year we were having, and he silenced me with a wave of his hand.

"We just want you to get better."

As my final Ampligen infusion neared, my attorney and I completed our plans. Hettie, Bill Christian, and I would all supply affidavits attesting to my improved health and function. We would somehow obtain the results from my treadmill and IQ tests at the close of the trial (I had managed to get the original baseline scores), and we would—if necessary—subpoena my doctor and the nurses who saw me regularly. We were not going to argue the point that HEM had broken its contractual promise; we were going to argue the case based on the ethics of ending a treatment that seemed to be helping me.

(Many months later, several patients from across the country joined together to sue HEM for breach of contract by not providing the drug as promised after the trial. They eventually were ordered to be treated with Ampligen for one year, pending a court date. Several of the patients later settled their suits for a six-month treatment extension.)

As the week of my final infusion arrived, I continued to show remarkable progress. I had gone out of town the previous weekend to moderate a meeting of news executives, and I'd managed to have a pretty good time. When I got home, just to prove I could do it, I hauled my lawn mower out of my storage shed and cut my back lawn. I hadn't even been in my back yard for more than a year! There was no way a judge could ignore this evidence, I reasoned.

I eagerly anticipated my final treadmill and IQ tests in Charlotte. Climbing on the treadmill, I felt the tingle of excitement that used to come from preparing for a lunchtime run at the fitness club. Of course, now I was wired with a half-dozen electrodes and a portable transmitter, and I had a scuba-like mask fitted tightly over my nose and into my mouth. Still, as I used to do on those midday jogs, I set a goal for myself. I knew I would reach it.

I stayed on the treadmill for six minutes longer than I'd been able to last time, and the computer indicated that my body was using oxygen much more efficiently than it had before I'd started on Ampligen. Though the test administrator didn't know how or why, he said that my individual cells were much healthier than they'd been at the beginning of the experiment. I was excited that I had more strong evidence for the judge, and I was even more excited that I seemed to be getting healthier.

The IQ tests turned out to be equally dramatic. At the beginning of the trial I'd been deep in the mind fog that's come to characterize the illness. My verbal IQ was 111—my performance score was a frightening 89. Now, six months later, my performance number had increased to 134, and my verbal IQ chimed in at 150. I had climbed out of the mind fog, and there was only one possible explanation—Ampligen.

My attorney consulted with a law firm in Charlotte, seeking to get an immediate hearing before a federal judge. As it turned out, we never needed the hearing.

I was driving to Charleston for a business meeting several hours after that final infusion. Between Florence and Charleston, there is a fifty-mile area where no cellular telephone service is available, and the moment I entered the Charleston cell, I dialed my voice-mail to check for messages. I immediately recognized the voice of Janie Warlick.

"Good news, Tim! HEM has declared you a significant responder. You'll start on open-label Ampligen next week—or as soon as they send it to me."

I was so excited I nearly drove off the road. I called Hettie, and we shared a prayer of thanksgiving. In our uphill struggle for my health, we'd just won a major battle.

Several weeks later, there was more good news. I received the itemized bill from my attorney. Though we had never gone to court, he and his co-counsel had done a lot of work on my case. They had even engaged the services of a firm in Charlotte, since neither of them were licensed in North Carolina. I opened the bill with some trepidation, for I had never paid for a lawyer's services out of my own pocket.

The charge was zero. The work had been done gratis. It was the most beautiful bill I'd ever received in my life.

I told Bill Christian about it and offered to return the check Diversified had given me.

"That's your money," he insisted. "We want you to have it. You'll need it one way or another."

I began open-label Ampligen a week later. But curiously, HEM stopped naming significant responders immediately after I and three others in Charlotte received the designation. Only a handful of other such patients were scattered around the country, and HEM put out the word that there would be no more. No one knew then—or knows now—why HEM did what it did. Every bit as mysterious is why I was chosen to stay on the drug and others who responded were not. Even now I am bothered by what I feel is akin to survivor's syndrome. I don't know why I was chosen and others weren't. I don't know why I was given a second chance.

Over the years since that cutoff, I have seen the toll that these decisions have taken. I know of one patient whose Ampligen treatment was suspended and who is not expected to live much longer. I know of another patient who was never a part of the trial but—according to her family—who became so despondent over what happened that she took her own life. I had no idea how serious this business of trying an experimental drug could be.

In the months after I started open-label Ampligen, many things concerning the drug happened in rapid succession—all of them disappointing. Most significantly, my condition began to deteriorate once again. The crash was back, worse than before. As the weeks after my six-month peak passed, I became sicker and sicker. By mid-summer, I was worse than I'd been at the beginning of the trial. My miracle cure—as everything else—had apparently failed me.

For the first time I began to seriously ponder the end of my career. My flying days had ended much earlier; I reasoned that my television days were numbered, too. Dr. Cheney guessed that the current dosage of Ampligen had helped me for a while, but increased amounts were needed to reverse this new and rapid decline.

The FDA denied HEM's application for a treatment (rather than an experimental) Ampligen protocol that would have allowed the drug to be used on hundreds of other patients around the country in varying doses. The agency took nearly a year to examine the data from our study before finally ordering another round of experimentation, and it also took nearly as long to approve an increase in my personal dosage. But by the time it granted that approval for a change in my dose, HEM had refused to grant Dr. Cheney's request for me to receive higher amounts of Ampligen. (I later learned that in the very first Ampligen tests in the Lake Tahoe area virtually all of the patients eventually crashed as I had, and they were immediately moved to a higher dosage. Once on the new dose, their conditions continued to improve.) Still, I counted my blessings that I was getting any Ampligen at all. I was one of only a handful of sufferers receiving the drug, and if it wasn't curing me, at least it was still giving me hope.

I would continue receiving Ampligen for two more years, through the summer of 1993. At that time, HEM announced it was ending all involvement with CFS patients. I suppose I knew the end was coming, and so I had prepared myself. I did feel a need to put the experience in perspective. After all, I'd practically been married to the drug, and then the marriage just ended.

I'd given a lot to Ampligen: forty-five thousand miles of driving for infusions, thirty-three months of my life, and nearly one thousand IV needles. But what had Ampligen given me?

I believe the drug was responsible for my brief "remission" after six months in the study. Beyond that, I felt no measurable improvement. In fact, for the last year on Ampligen, I actually seemed to be doing worse immediately after my infusions. I was having stomach and gall bladder problems, too, which eventually landed me in the hospital for surgery. Was it the drug? Was it CFS? No one can tell me.

During that final year, finding a vein in which to insert an IV had become an ordeal. Sometimes the effort took nearly an hour and required five or six attempts. I would soak my arms in hot water to get my veins to stand up, but even that trick lost its effectiveness. I could have had a catheter inserted permanently allowing direct access to a major vein in my chest, but I decided against that. Several CFS patients (not on Ampligen) who had done this had seen their catheters became infected because of their weakened immune systems. A few of them died.

So I stuck with the needles and I stuck with the Ampligen. I was the final Charlotte patient to receive infusions, and even though those last few bottles held no promise of health benefit, I took the medicine that I'd fought so hard to get. I tell people I rode that train as far as it would go. I look back on the trip with disappointment and lingering questions, but not with regret.

Somewhere in the files of the FDA and HEM may rest an answer to the question of what good Ampligen did for me. However, no one is sharing the answer with me. While I got the IQ scores and treadmill test results, I was never shown any significant data on cellular tests. Every eight weeks, my blood samples were sent to sophisticated labs in several states. I saw only the routine test results, things like white blood cell counts, liver enzymes, and iron levels. I was told that scientists were looking at a specific antiviral mechanism in my immune system, but I never did learn what they found. I deserve to know.

When I speak to CFS support groups, I am often asked about Ampligen. Thousands of people are pinning their hopes of a normal life on the drug, despite the disrupted trials and the rocky approval process. What do I tell these people about a drug that was so much a part of my life yet left so many questions unanswered? I choose my words carefully, and when I share my Ampligen experience, I always begin like this: "We know that a person can survive as long as a month without food, three or four days without water, and even a couple of minutes without oxygen. But I am convinced that living without hope is impossible, even for a moment. During a very critical period of my life, Ampligen provided the hope that kept me going."

I am convinced that with hope, even the darkest circumstances can appear survivable. So when it comes to Ampligen, I resist the urge to tell other patients merely of my doubts. Instead, I try to recall the determination with which I fought to get into the study protocol. I try to recall that for months I kept trying, kept hanging on, kept hoping. I try to recall that at a time when I had so little to look forward to, the prospect of receiving Ampligen kept me thinking about tomorrow. And I always tell them about how good I was feeling after six months—I always talk about the day I mowed the lawn.

There's another story I tell them involving one of the most bizarre symptoms associated with CFS. Incredibly, as many as fifteen percent of CFS patients see their fingerprints fade away. That's what happened to me in the second year of my illness. Soon after, I heard of a researcher who was looking at the phenomenon, and I asked to be a part of his small, informal study.

What this researcher told me—it has yet to be published—was amazing. Of all the patients in the study, I was the only one showing evidence that something was working to stop the tissue damage. The only reason I could imagine for this was Ampligen.

If some sort of viral agent were destroying the tissue in my fingers and Ampligen was working to stop that, perhaps Ampligen was doing me some good. I could only hope that what was happening in my fingertips was happening throughout the rest of my body.

Forty-five thousand miles, thirty-three months, a thousand needles. I suppose that is not too great a price to pay for what may be the most important medicine of all: hope.

11

THE SOCIAL SQUEEZE

Dim lighting from the candles created a warm feeling as I slid quietly into the pew. It was 7:29 P.M. on Christmas Eve, 1991, and the special service at our church, one of the local Methodist congregations, was about to begin. The organ prelude was ending, and the pastor stood ready to approach his pulpit.

I had decided only fifteen minutes earlier to attend this service. Three years had passed since I had become ill, and it had been three years since I'd last been in this beautiful sanctuary. Lying on the sofa at home, I had remembered the special holiday service and what it had once meant to me, and I'd quickly changed into a fresh shirt and told Hettie I was going.

This church had been at the center of our lives for the first several years we were in South Carolina. The people in the congregation had been our family, and the sanctuary had been a kind of home for us. In a sense, we had grown up as a couple at the church.

I looked around in the candlelight, revisiting those times in my mind. I had been an usher here, a member of the administrative board, a Sunday School teacher. On Sunday mornings, I would stand at the pulpit and welcome visitors, calling their names and instructing the congregation to make them feel welcome. My last duty at the church, just before I became ill, had been to supervise the design and installation of a new audio system, and I had never returned to hear the results. As the pastor opened the Christmas Eve service with a traditional prayer, I smiled at the richness of his voice filling the worship hall. The "new" sound system was an achievement I had forgotten until I spotted the speakers suspended below the arched ceiling. I was pleased at its performance.

Being a Sunday School teacher, welcoming visitors, seating parishioners, and sitting on the church board were all facts I knew; they were not experiences I recalled. Such is the effect of CFS on the mind. Facts can survive, memories often do not. And so as I tried to blend into this congregation for the first time in thirty-six months, I knew that this place and these people had at one time meant a great deal to me, but I could not recall those feelings. The chasm between knowing and remembering cannot be imagined until it is experienced.

The holiday service was brief, and the congregation closed the program by passing candles from one to another and singing "Silent Night." It was good to be in church again. I was pleased that a window of wellness had opened for me this night, and that I had taken advantage of it to make my way to church as I had the very first time I had entered it: as a faceless visitor, trying to slip in and out undetected. Or so I hoped.

As I unlocked my car door to head home, a voice called out from behind.

"Tim! Tim Kenny! Merry Christmas!"

I turned and looked into what seemed to be a familiar face, but I couldn't recall the man's name. His two young children were with him, wearing their holiday outfits and bright holiday smiles. I must have known them as babies, but I struggled without success to remember their names.

Another person called to me and shook my hand vigorously.

Someone else hugged me, saying it was good to see me in church again.

I stumbled to make polite conversation, wishing my greeters a happy holiday, vaguely recalling how close we had once been. We had shared suppers and meetings, and prayers by the hundreds. I had seen them start families, buy homes, change jobs, baptize children. Now, just three years later, I couldn't even remember their names.

They smiled broadly at me, asking about Hettie, inviting me to come back. It was like watching a foreign movie dubbed into

English; I understood their words, but everything else seemed to be from another world.

"We sure hope you come back again . . . we've missed you!" I heard someone say.

I smiled and thanked them, then got into my car and started it up.

"Thank you . . . thank you very much," I managed as I backed the car out, my headlights sweeping across this handful of nice people.

"Merry Christmas to you, too," I said through the window.

The drive home took less than two minutes, yet I felt as if I were on a journey through time. These people with whom I'd once been so close had acted as if I had moved to some faraway continent and had returned for just a short visit. The irony washed over me as I turned into my driveway, my car's heater never having had a chance to warm my chilled feet. I hadn't moved anywhere; I was where I'd always been—nine-tenths of a mile from the church. But that night, the distance seemed a million times greater. I just kept wondering that if these fine people had cared so much, where had they been for the past three years?

I have lost a lot to this illness, but there are times when I think I miss my friends more than anything else. When people go through long periods of isolation, such as CFS imposes, something happens to their interpersonal skills. I could have responded more to the few people who were attempting to reach out to me, but I had forgotten how to be a friend myself. It will take time and effort on my part to repair these relationships, and understanding on the part of the friends I have retained. Friends have to recognize that if I don't return their calls immediately, it's not because I'm uncaring, but rather that I'm too sick to talk. And if they see me and I'm intolerable, it's because they've hit me on a bad day when I feel absolutely terrible. During the period when I was declining so rapidly and seeing so much of my life slip away, I said and did things that I should not have. I just hope that I can explain it all now that I understand it myself.

I was a shy youngster with an inferiority complex. My early

group of friends had been small, confined mostly to a buddy who lived across the street from me and played on the same Little League team. Many years later, as I began to achieve some success in broadcasting, I started to make friends and spend more time in social situations. More than just a prerequisite for my position, being with friends became a treat I had not known before. I went from being a wallflower as a child to enjoying center stage in my twenties. The experience was both liberating and fulfilling.

I did all kinds of things with my friends—from flying airplanes to playing tennis to having a beer after the eleven o'clock news. In my mid- and late-twenties, I was experiencing socially what most people experienced during college. I had married early, and was busy earning a living when my contemporaries were throwing Frisbees and chugging beer. Now I'd discovered the simple fun of having a good time with other people. It was one of the most enjoyable periods of my life, and it ended when I got sick.

For one thing, no one knew what was wrong with me. I declined invitations to parties and tennis games, I faded after one beer, I couldn't stand loud music. Sometimes I was moody and bitter, and I rarely laughed as I used to. I appeared to be consumed with work, struggling to do my job and with little energy for anything else.

I quit going to movies; I quit going out to lunch or dinner. My flying buddies wondered why they never saw me at the airport anymore. Church friends later told me they thought I was withdrawing. Family visits or get-togethers of any sort were all but out of the question. People stopped dropping by after they found me propped up on the sofa looking pale and wasted. We no longer got invited to other people's homes.

My final year at WPDE, I struggled against my protesting body to make a thirty-minute appearance at our company Christmas party. It was all I could manage, and I considered it a superhuman effort. I noticed that some of the other department heads were talking about my "attitude." I skipped our station's last two summer picnics, only to hear that I was becoming snobby or antisocial or— worst of all—that I didn't care about my job anymore and I was cutting corners.

I didn't go to fireworks shows on Independence Day, I didn't go Christmas shopping, I didn't show up at Super Bowl parties.

One friend summed it up well: "Get with the program, Tim," she said. "You're really not much fun anymore."

All of that was before my diagnosis. After the terrible label of CFS was attached to my behavior, most people gave up even trying to get me to do anything. I was tired and burned out, they reasoned, and I surely wasn't the life of any parties anymore. It was better just to leave Tim alone.

In defense of my friends and colleagues, I am certain that some of my actions drove them away as much as my physical appearance and limitations did. I *was* angry and bitter—I was watching my happy new life slipping away. I *was* moody—I was cheerful when I felt good, foul-tempered when I was feeling my worst, and my symptoms could come and go quickly. My friend was right; I wasn't much fun anymore.

And so, one by one, my friends did a slow fade. I still saw them at work or in other settings, but our time together wasn't as it used to be. The hours of laughing and carrying on were over for me. I couldn't keep up, and I couldn't explain why. What little extra energy I could summon was expended on the twice-weekly trips to Charlotte.

At first, several friends offered to make that journey with me to find out what I was going through. Only a couple ever did, and I'm sure the sight of their buddy hooked up to an IV, in pain, and looking scared and helpless, was not pleasant. Others kept promising to come someday, making empty offers to help me with the drive. I longed for their company, especially in the months after I stopped working, but these people had exciting lives to lead and I knew that other commitments would win out. In addition, being around someone who was once so full of life and is now in such a fragile state must be very uncomfortable—it reminds the well friends of their own mortality.

Chronic illness, death, or other tragedies that befall some people make bystanders uncomfortable. They don't know what to say or how to act when faced with someone who has been crippled, someone who has suffered a great loss, someone with CFS. So they stay away.

I recently heard that someone I worked with had lost his mother just a few days earlier, and I called his workplace to find out more. No one there could provide details. "I don't think he wants anyone to know," one of the people told me.

I called this fellow at home anyway. Despite his co-workers' perceptions, we had a wonderful conversation about his mother. He told me about his mother, about how she had lived and how she had died, and he talked practically nonstop for thirty minutes. I asked if there was anything I could do for him, and he said that there was. (Imagine—me getting the chance to do something for someone else for a change!) I was glad that he accepted my offer, and I was glad that I was able to accomplish the task.

"I'm surprised no one at work told me anything like this," I mentioned.

"Yeah, I was expecting to hear from some people there, but I haven't yet," he said.

Too often, that's how it goes. Friends made uncomfortable by tragedy miss the opportunity to do good—for themselves as well as for those suffering loss. We should all make the effort to step across the line of discomfort, reach out to someone who might be alone in their circumstances. It can make a world of difference for the person in need and might really make you feel good about yourself.

In talking to other CFS patients, I hear much the same story. Marriages and engagements have been destroyed and families have fallen apart. Patients have even attempted suicide to escape the loneliness. Tragically, many have succeeded.

Occasionally, there are stories that bring back hope. The crisis brings some families closer together, actually strengthening the relationships. Some friendships—though very few—flourish under the pressure of CFS. Most patients I know spend the majority of their time alone or with one or two devoted friends or family members. Their phones rarely ring; there is rarely a knock at the door.

Certainly it is not pleasant to see someone you care about going through an experience as consuming, devastating, and mysterious as serious illness. But I never accepted that as a reason for abandoning someone, and I still don't. Ignorance and fear are simply not good enough excuses for turning your back on other people when they need you most.

On the rare occasions that I have had the courage to discuss this with former friends, their response has usually been, "I just figured if you needed something, you'd call. I didn't want to bother you." They didn't think that in the lonely months after CFS took my health, my career, and most of my relationships, I would long to be "bothered." However, when I mentioned this to my friends, they would withdraw even more. No one likes to be told he is inadequate.

"Hey, man, *you're* the one who drove me away."

"I just couldn't believe how you treated me that one time when you were. . . ." (Fill in the episode.)

"You really hurt my feelings when you said that I never called you, so I just quit doing it."

"So-and-so told me you said I wasn't being the kind of friend I used to. Thanks for nothing. Why do you think I never came around!"

"I just gave up trying to figure you out."

And so people who once occupied major roles in my life are now little more than memories. They don't call or write; I hear about them only through mutual friends. I miss them. About once a month I get a call from an old colleague. After the pleasantries, the caller normally says something like this:

"Tim, I'm calling for two reasons. First, I wanted to see how you're doing. Second, I wondered if I could put you down as a job reference . . ."

I do like hearing from these people, so I generally don't get too riled about this. I just wish they'd be honest. It would be so much simpler for them, and more appealing to me. It could be something as plain as "I've been so busy I haven't thought about calling you lately, but I thought you'd be a good person to list as a job reference so I wanted to check with you." I retain my dignity, and there's no embarrassment for the caller or for me.

Thankfully, there have been a few wonderful exceptions. My wife, Hettie, tops the list.

She was eighteen when we stood in a Methodist church in rural Pennsylvania on a steamy August evening and uttered those words, "For better or for worse, for richer or poorer, in sickness and in health. . . ." For most newlyweds, this vow is never tested in the negative. No one would blame Hettie for abandoning those vows, considering all that my illness has robbed her of, but she has never wavered in the duty she took on that day. There have been terrible times, month after month filled with hopeless wondering, wasted holidays, spoiled vacations, and miserable week after miserable week, but Hettie has kept her promise to me. We are closer today than ever before, and I pray for my health to return so that I can repay her in the years to come.

Some family members, after a few uncertain months, have also become closer to me despite our geographical separation. And there are still a handful of people—I call them my Hall of Fame— who have remained friends through all of this. There's is an invaluable loyalty. They are an interesting cross-section of the world I lived in: a handful of TV news people, a couple of acquaintances from ABC, two guys who design race car decals for NASCAR, some broadcasting engineers, and a couple of folks who really don't fit into any particular category except that they're around when I call them. These are very special people.

I have also made new friends through this illness—patients like me who know the pain I feel and understand the destruction caused by CFS. I have made friends with people like Janie Warlick and others in Dr. Cheney's office, as well as with some people within the CFS movement.

But for those who remain close from years past, coping with the strains caused by this illness does not make fertile ground for planting seeds for future experiences together.

One such friend, now in another state, told me for months about how he would be spending an upcoming vacation in the Carolinas, and how we would get together for some good times. The good times, it turned out, were at the airport near my home where he was changing planes on the way home from his vacation, spent with other, more mobile, friends.

I understood why that was as we were walking through the airport terminal in the few minutes we had between his flights.

"I guess this is the last time I'll be seeing you for a while," I said.

"I'll be back in Myrtle Beach for a bachelor party in a couple of months," he said. "Maybe I can stop at your house on the way. I'm sure you won't feel like coming."

"Please don't assume that," I said. "Invite me. If I'm able, I'll come. If I'm not, at least I'll know you wanted me there."

A broad smile crossed my buddy's face.

"Yeah, we sure had some good times!" he mused. "It would be great to do it one more time before I get married."

He put his hand on my shoulder as he said those words, and I wanted to find a way to bottle the feeling that passed over me at that instant. Here was a friend who was trying to adapt and respond to my situation, even though our lives were now so totally different. He was a well-known television personality in another city, embarking on a new life and great career success at the same time I was sitting in my house waiting for the mail to come. Yet in that instant, he reached out to understand me and make an effort to include me in his life.

We laughed about the good times we'd shared in years passed, and swapped a few old war stories. In a few moments he disappeared into the crowd of passengers heading toward their planes, giving me one more smile and wave.

"I'll let you know about the party," he said as he turned away. "I hope you can be there!"

I felt good that evening, appreciating that this dear friend was trying hard to include me in his life.

It will probably come as no surprise that I never made it to that bachelor party. The invitation was repeated once or twice after the airport meeting, always in general terms, always leaving me feeling that my buddy didn't really know how to handle the situation. Bachelor parties are usually loud and boisterous, with lots of drinking and carrying on. My friend was caught in a difficult dilemma—inviting me to an event that I was really not up to, or making me feel left out.

He did the best he could, and I appreciate it. The lesson to everyone who has an ill friend or family member should be to at least make the effort, as my buddy did. At least ask, at least try to include us. That attempt means more than you'll ever know. And maybe someday, we'll actually feel up to accepting the invitation.

Thinking now of my buddy, his vacation, and the bachelor party, I am touched by the difficulty of his predicament and the attempt he made to reach out to me. Sometimes in the bitter social squeeze of this miserably misunderstood illness, a few sweet drops emerge.

Thanks, friend.

12

THE PSYCHOLOGY OF QUITTING

In August 1991, the time had come when I needed to mark the end of my career at WPDE. Deep down I knew it was a necessary step, but I couldn't pull the plug myself. I had spent so much of my life overcoming challenges and exceeding expectations that I couldn't conceive of voluntarily stopping. I needed someone to make this decision for me.

On August 15, Hettie and I met with Dr. Cheney to evaluate my prognosis. My health had been deteriorating, and there was simply no reason for optimism. I'd done everything I could to keep working: I was seeing the top CFS clinician in the world, I was on the only experimental drug approved for study on CFS patients, and I'd learned all I could about the illness. A handful of government agencies and experts from nearly a dozen major medical universities had studied some parts of me. Yet despite all this, the bottom line was simple: I was getting worse, not better.

I asked Dr. Cheney the question that had been on my mind for months, hoping that perhaps he would make the painful decision one way or another for me. My heart said one thing; my body and mind were telling me quite another.

"What about keeping working . . . maintaining ten- and twelve-hour days?" I'd asked. "What impact is that likely to have on my chances of getting better?"

Dr. Cheney did not hesitate. "Clearly, you've suffered some serious brain damage. That's obvious."

Thinking of the IQ tests, the memory problems, and other anecdotal episodes like the mysterious car accident, I had to agree.

I didn't have access to the technical knowledge that Dr. Cheney did, but I was living proof that my brain was not what it had been a few years earlier.

"The thing that I keep thinking," he continued, "is that the more you force yourself to do things now, the more brain damage you are probably causing. *Rest* is too simple a word, but you've got to take it much easier. At this rate," he said, pointing to my chart for emphasis, "I could well be looking at an Alzheimer's patient by the time you're forty. We've seen this kind of damage before, but never in people so young. There's just no way to know. . . ." His voice trailed off.

I thought for a moment about what he said. "I'm not trying to put words in your mouth," I said, "but are you telling me that if I don't stop working now, I may never be able to get well . . . I might never work again?"

Cheney nodded.

"If things continue as they are now, that's the most likely case," he said. "I know it's a hard thing to do, but when you think of an entire lifetime, a few years is a small price to pay to get well."

I tried to hide my disappointment, though I had entered this meeting expecting exactly what Dr. Cheney had just said. My own experience was screaming to me that the time had come to step down from my job. Logic told me it made sense, but my emotions weren't listening. I had worked like a maniac to get to where I was. A simple sabbatical didn't work in my industry; taking a few years to mend would most likely mean the end of my career in television. Without that career, life didn't seem worth living.

A friend put it well a day later: "I know it's killing you to keep working," he said. "I can see it in your eyes, I can see it in your steps, I can hear it in your voice. But quitting working . . . that might kill you even faster."

In Dr. Cheney's office, Hettie and I exchanged glances. We'd danced around the subject of my leaving my job over the past year, and we'd spent more and more time discussing it recently.

"Are you saying I'm eligible for total disability? Am I *really* sick?" I asked.

"No question," he said, again pointing to my chart. "The evidence is all there. You're a very sick person."

We ended the meeting with the three of us all agreeing that the time indeed had come for me to stop. Dr. Cheney would draft a letter to my company and fax it to me the next day.

When Dr. Cheney's letter came, I carried it around tightly wrapped in my fist. Before showing it to anyone, I needed practical answers to some very important questions. I closed the door to my office and placed a call to our corporate headquarters in Portland, Maine.

In a moment, Liz Crosby, our human resources manager, answered her phone. Liz knew about my condition, but as with most people in the corporation, I'd hidden its severity from her. I hoped to be in line for a promotion someday soon to general manager, where I would be running an entire station, and I'd tried to hide the worst of my situation from the people in Portland, not wanting to exclude myself from the selection process.

I'd known Liz since I joined the company. I had become her local correspondent for the corporate newsletter, and she'd dealt with my hectic schedule by stretching deadlines for me for the previous five years. On my annual vacations to Maine, I'd always spend a little time with Liz, and whenever she came to Florence we managed a brief private visit, too. In the world of big business, Liz and Diversified Communications are the antithesis to the uncaring, inhuman corporate attitude. Liz, I later learned, had played a large role in the special bonus check I'd received to fight the Ampligen battle. Such actions were typical of the caring and warmth that flowed southward from Portland to our little TV station in South Carolina.

I remember that in the hours just before Hurricane Hugo hit, we received a call from company president George Anderson: "Forget about profits; forget about making money. Serve the viewers as best you can, but above all, don't risk your lives."

Such was the attitude that existed in my company, and I knew that no matter how severely my situation had deteriorated, these people cared about me as a person first.

I made small talk with Liz before shifting to the purpose of my call.

"Liz, I can't name names right now, but I have an employee I'd like to ask you about."

It was not unusual for us to have such conversations. Diversified was a self-insured corporation, and I often spoke to Liz on behalf of anonymous employees with sensitive questions relating to our health insurance program.

"Sure, go ahead," Liz urged me.

"Well, I'd like to know about long-term disability insurance," I said with a measured effort to sound disinterested. "Can you tell me how it works, how much it pays, and how it impacts the company?"

The last part of the question was important to me, for though I had agreed with Dr. Cheney that I had to stop working, I wouldn't do it if the move would hurt our small corporation. Such kindness and compassion as Diversified's breeds tremendous loyalty from employees, and I didn't want to become a financial burden to this great company.

Liz explained the disability process. Diversified maintained all pay and benefits for six months after the disability began. Then the employee would be officially terminated—Liz never actually said *terminated*, calling it instead the "T word,"—and then our private disability carrier would pay a monthly benefit equal to sixty percent of the person's salary. Liz said they'd only gone through this process one or twice before, but that it was fairly routine. The only cash outlay by the company, she told me, was the six-month salary continuation, designed to get the employee through the insurance company's deductible period. After that, the employee was free to maintain his or her health insurance policy (previously a paid company benefit) for about two hundred dollars a month.

I now had what I needed to know about the business aspect of quitting my job. I thanked Liz for the information, and hung up.

For several minutes after my conversation with Liz, I kept denying what I knew I had to do right then. I had never quit anything in my life; I'd never met a foe that demanded my surrender. My life had been an uphill battle from the start (I nearly died before I was born), and I was used to fighting difficult odds. But CFS was an unprecedented obstacle in my life. Sheer will and determination seemed no match for what it had done to me.

I sat in my closed office, my head bowed in my hands, not answering my telephone page, ignoring the knocks at my door.

I looked again at Dr. Cheney's disability letter. If I just tore it up, I reasoned from the deep pit of denial, all of this would go away. But I knew better. I had run from CFS for two years. I had run, and it kept finding me. Ripping the letter to pieces wouldn't change the facts as I'd come to see them. I had run out of options.

Still, I decided to spend the weekend thinking about everything before I finally talked to my company. My friend Bill Christian had been transferred to another station only weeks before, and we had a young new general manager, Mike Reed. The new company president, Garry Ritchie, had called me just two weeks earlier with the message *we need you, Tim, now more than ever.* My best friend, Tom Sorrells, the meteorologist, had also left a few months earlier for a bigger job in Columbus, Ohio. While the departures of Bill and Tommy did mean that the station needed me more than ever, they also took away two of the biggest reasons I had hung on so long. Working with these two guys was a dream come true. We had been a great team, but now only I remained.

I would take the weekend and think this over. But I had one more bit of business to take care of.

I hit the redial button on my phone, and got Liz on the phone again.

"Liz," I began, "I've known you too long to lie to you. Can you take off your company hat and be my friend for a moment?"

"Sure, Tim."

"There is no hypothetical employee," I confessed. "I was asking you about me."

"I know," Liz responded. "I'm glad you called back. What can I do to help?"

I told Liz that more than anything I just wanted some personal advice, some help making this painful decision. As it turned out, Liz was the perfect person to ask.

She told me about her husband, diagnosed one summer with cancer. Several weeks later, after desperate surgery, he died. It had all been so sudden there were never any options to consider—there'd been no second chance for him.

"We'd have given anything for a second chance back then, Tim," she said. "Anything. But we didn't get one. Maybe this is your second chance . . . maybe you'll get through this if you follow the doctor's advice. Maybe you'll be back someday."

The profoundness of her statement was irrefutable. In that perspective, maybe I was making too big a deal out of this whole thing. She was right. If I were to get a second chance, it would come only from stepping back from my career and allowing my body to heal. I could now view the disability decision in a new light—as a second chance and not a final option.

I thanked Liz for her wonderful counsel and asked that she not discuss our conversation with any of the corporate officers. Liz abides by honesty. "I won't go in there and tell them we talked about this," she promised. "But if someone comes into my office and asks me if Tim Kenny just called about disability, I'll have to tell them, okay?"

I smiled at her caring. That was more than fair. For the first time, I began to finally believe that I was going to leave.

I looked around my office, filled with memorabilia. "It's been a helluva run," I'd tell a friend a few days later, "But it's time to cancel this show forever."

I hid the letter in my desk drawer and immersed myself in the Friday night news. Hurricane Bob was a potential threat to our coastline. Hurricane coverage was my specialty; Bob provided a harmless distraction as it skirted past our shore and back out to sea over the weekend.

Monday morning I made my way to Mike Reed's office. I had known Mike since the day he'd started at WPDE nearly a decade before. We'd come up through our company's ranks together, and before this day I had actually believed we'd be counterparts sometime, him running WPDE, me heading up another of our group's stations. As I asked him to come to my office that morning, I knew my vision of being a general manager would never come to pass.

When Mike got to my office, I showed him Dr. Cheney's letter. Then I presented him with two documents of my own, both born out of my denial over what was happening. The first memo absolved Diversified and WPDE of any responsibility for my health from that day forward, should I stay on the job. The second memo presented Mike with three options: Allow me to keep my job on a part-time basis, allow me to stay in the position until a replacement was found, and accept Dr. Cheney's verdict. To the very end, I wanted other people to make this painful decision for me.

Mike was stunned. He'd been at the station all weekend and had seen me orchestrate the Hurricane Bob coverage. Like everyone else I worked with, he knew I was sick, but he had no idea it was serious. And he'd been the general manager for only two months before I—the manager of his largest and most visible department—had confronted him with this problem.

I lobbied Mike to consider my first two options, the part-time work or staying on the job until a replacement could be found. Cheney's letter didn't address either of those possibilities, I knew, but I was still trying hard to put off the inevitable.

Mike shook his head.

"According to this, you need to stop working right away," he said. Then he read the letter again. Finally, he paused and looked up. The color had been drained from his face and he spoke slowly.

"Let me talk to Portland about this."

"Sure . . . of course," I stammered. I still couldn't believe we were talking about my departure. It just didn't seem possible. But the look on Mike's face told me what any reasonable person would have been able to tell from reading the letter; Dr. Cheney wasn't suggesting any options, any delays, any part-time positions. He was talking about *right now*.

Mike disappeared down the hall toward his own office, and I poured myself into another Monday morning in the TV news business. That night I dragged myself home, exhausted and disoriented, and for the first time in my life feeling that my career was no longer in my hands.

* * *

The next morning I was back at my desk acting as if nothing had happened. I had told no one other than Mike about the disability letter, and I figured I'd just keep working until someone told me to quit. I didn't have long to wait.

At about 11:20, a half-hour before I was to leave for my Ampligen infusion, Mike appeared in my office. Closing the doors, he drew a chair near to my desk and sat down.

"This is hard," he began, his voice almost hoarse as he spoke the words.

I put down my pen and nodded.

"I talked to everybody in Portland and I talked to your doctor," Mike said. "We really don't have any option . . ."

"But I suggested a couple of things in my memo," I interrupted.

"Tim, this letter from your doctor is dated Friday," he said. "We're liable for your working this weekend, yesterday . . . we're even liable that you're here right now. We just don't have any choice but to comply with what Dr. Cheney says."

I had entered that television station nearly a decade earlier, young, inexperienced, and naive. But now I was a professional in every sense. I reached deep within that part of my character and began to speak, sensing Mike had said all he could.

"I understand," I remember saying softly. I pushed slowly back from my desk, took a deep breath, and asked the question that sounded as if it were coming from someone else.

"How soon do you want me out?"

Mike looked at the floor, and then back up at me.

"Right now," he said. "I'd like to call a department head meeting and announce it immediately."

No—this was how they fired people. I wasn't going to leave this way. I had another idea. I wanted to tell my staff first; they'd been with me through thick and thin, they came first. We could overlook protocol this one time and bypass the other managers. I asked Mike if I might have a staff meeting immediately after the six o'clock news to tell my own department. We would make a formal announcement to everyone else in the morning.

Mike agreed to my request, and I stood to shake his hand. Instead, he embraced me silently before slipping out of my office and disappearing down the hall.

I looked at my watch. I had to leave for Charlotte in ten minutes—the Ampligen was waiting. Calling to my executive producer, I told him to announce a mandatory news meeting at 6:40 that evening. When he asked me why we were having the sudden meeting, I told him he'd find out with everyone else.

"You're not going to . . . ?" he began, but I cut him off.

"Tonight, Robert," I said. "You'll find out tonight."

Janie Warlick was especially sensitive to me that afternoon at Dr. Cheney's office, asking again and again if I were doing okay. I had told her that this was to be my last day on the job, and she seemed very concerned.

"I'm fine," I kept saying when she'd ask. It was a lie, and we both knew it.

When my infusion was nearly completed, Janie came to me and leaned close. "We're concerned about you," she said softly. I assumed that "we" was Janie and the other nurse I knew well, Sheryl Autry.

As the final drops from the Ampligen bottle snaked their way through the IV, Janie told me about a psychologist in the building just across the parking lot from Dr. Cheney's office. Dr. Wayne Robertson had seen many patients whose lives had been shattered by diseases like CFS and MS. She thought it would be a good idea for me to pay him a visit. Looking back on that suggestion, I realize it was one of the most insightful and courageous things another person has ever done for me.

I checked my watch. I could see this guy if I went over right now, but any later and I wouldn't make it back to the TV station for my meeting.

She disappeared to make a call, returning shortly with Dr. Robertson's office address written on a scrap of paper.

"He's expecting you right now," she said.

What the heck, I thought. Maybe she knew something I

didn't. As it turned out, her intervention may well have saved my life.

I found Dr. Robertson to be kind and soft-spoken, and he listened to me recite a quick history of the events leading up to that day. He talked to me about the meeting I was about to have with my staff and about some of the emotions I was likely to experience. It was a simple and nonthreatening session. When he suggested I come back the following week and tell him how I was doing, I shrugged my shoulders and agreed.

"Sure," I said. "I'll probably really need to talk to someone after a week without working."

In the elevator outside Dr. Robertson's office, the reality of the day finally began to sink in. I was about to pull the plug on my job, my career, my identity, my paycheck, my proof that I was somebody. There would be no more hurricanes, no more meetings in Hollywood, no more young superstar journalists to hire and train, no more employees to surround myself with as an extended family. Though I had suspected for months that this day would come, and though the wheels had been in motion since the meeting with Dr. Cheney the previous week, my denial reflex had kept me from confronting the reality of it all. As the elevator doors slid open on the ground floor, I looked out at a world that was suddenly very different.

For once, I was thankful that the drive back to my office took more than two hours. I needed the time to absorb this all and prepare for telling my staff goodbye. I wanted them to know how much they meant to me and how much I'd miss them, but I didn't want to become too emotional. And of course I knew they'd be worried about their own jobs—change brings great insecurity in television—and I would do whatever I could to lay their fears to rest.

Leaving Charlotte behind me that afternoon, I slid my favorite Jimmy Buffett tape into the car stereo. The words to my choice Buffett song, "Trying to Reason with Hurricane Season," seemed that day to have been written for my life, for that very hour:

Now I must confess
I could use some rest.
I can't run at this pace very long.
Yes it's quite insane,
I think it hurts my brain.
But it cleans me out and then I can go on.

I played the song again and again as I got closer to Florence. Its relevance and meaning grew with each reprise.

I arrived at WPDE as the six o'clock news was ending. My Myrtle Beach staff had driven to the main studio for this mysterious meeting, and their infrequent presence always meant a little extra rowdiness in the hallways and the newsroom. As I opened the door from the parking lot, I could hear them all carrying on.

No one knew why I had called this meeting so suddenly. In my tenure as news director, I'd tried to keep total staff meetings to a minimum; it was such a hassle trying to get everyone together. That practice had made tonight's meeting even more of a question mark, and the noisy kidding I heard in the hallways was just one way they were trying to alleviate their apprehension.

As soon as I could, I gathered the twenty-four curious faces into our station's large conference room, and without pausing long enough to allow them to wonder what was happening, I announced my departure. I recited the Jimmy Buffett lyrics to them, and told them that I had to rest or I could never come back. Whatever this was, it was hurting my brain.

The room full of people fell silent. I stood at the head of the table, not knowing quite what to do next.

"I just want you all to know how much you mean to me . . . how proud I am of you," I said. "I don't think there's a better TV news team in any market in America. This is the hardest goodbye I could ever imagine, but I'm leaving knowing that I've helped bring together a great bunch of people, and you've all helped to make me look good."

I looked around the room and studied them all. There was Amanda, whom I had hired out of college and sent to journalistic boot camp at our Myrtle Beach bureau in the weeks following Hugo. There was David, once an awkward kid who had turned into one of my most valuable players. There was Clay, whom I'd known for years. Poor Clay, I thought of this long-time WPDE employee, he's about to get *another* news director. He'd been through many transitions already.

I looked at Glenn and Sherena, a husband and wife who had been out of work when I made them my morning anchor team and allowed Sherena to develop weather skills that would eventually take her to one of the largest markets and best TV stations in the country. I saw Bob, the man whom I'd replaced as news director two years earlier. He had weathered that like a pro, and he was the market's top anchorman. I looked at Kevan, whom I'd just hired from The Weather Channel to replace Tom Sorrells. I'd promised Kevan a news director who would be beside him every step of the way, and now I was breaking that promise.

Bo, my sportscaster, was another success story. I had chosen him right out of college, spotting his raw talent in the first few seconds of his resume tape. I loved just sitting around and talking sports with Bo, but it would happen no more.

Mick was my chief photographer, perhaps my most loyal employee. We had endured Myrtle Beach "hell weeks" together, and we had a special respect and admiration for each other. It hurt to know we would never work together that way again.

Shaunya, my anchorwoman, had silent tears in her eyes, and they were becoming contagious. I had hired Shaun from a terrible situation in a smaller market, and she had flourished at our anchor desk. We had shared many deep and personal discussions in this very conference room, but like all of my other memories of this wonderful group, it would be no more.

There were more than a dozen others, all of them special to me. I would miss them all.

They looked at me standing there, trying to think of what to say next as I played through those memories. By now, I was blinking back tears of my own.

"I had wanted to go around the room and tell my favorite story about each of you," I said. "That's how I wanted to end this meeting, with laughs and funny stories. But I think I'm becoming too emotional . . . I don't think I can do it."

I turned to them, disappointed that I had failed them by having to leave, and disappointed that I had failed to do what I'd planned in that meeting.

And then, after only a moment of silence, my noon anchorman, Wayne, spoke up.

"Well, if you can't tell how you feel about us," he said, "we'll tell you how we feel about you."

With that, Wayne rose to his feet and began to clap, slowly at first, and then faster. Then the rest of the crew were on their feet, joining Wayne in the first and only standing ovation I have ever gotten in my life. It was the most moving tribute any boss could have asked for, and I have replayed it in my mind a thousand times since.

As their applause continued, the tears I'd been blinking back appeared in full force. Most of us were crying now, and none of us were ashamed. Finally, I motioned for the clapping to stop.

"Aw, what the heck," I managed to say with a laugh. "I can't let Wayne get the last word! I'll tell my stories after all."

And so I spent the next fifteen minutes going from person to person, telling story after story, each one ending with a preplanned punchline that brought bursts of laughter from everyone in the room. We'd sure racked up some great memories, more than enough to fill any person's career highlight reel a dozen times over. I am so thankful that Wayne's act gave me the courage to say goodbye the way I'd planned.

"In my last official act as your boss, I want to demand that you all have successful careers and continue to make me proud," I said finally. "And I declare this meeting officially over."

I quickly left the room and adjourned to my office, hoping that I could keep my composure now. But one by one my staff members came in to share their individual farewells, and by the time they finished we were all crying. (I didn't see the eleven o'clock news that night, but I'm sure every person who appeared on camera must have had bloodshot eyes.)

With the last goodbye over, I quietly turned off my office lights and closed the door behind me, slipping down the hall and out into the parking lot.

Hettie was waiting for me when I got home. I really couldn't say anything, and she really didn't ask. She just held me as I shook my head in disbelief over what had happened.

The next morning I arrived at my office thirty minutes early, wearing my finest suit, determined to leave with the professional manner I'd learned and honed while at WPDE.

The department head meeting began promptly at 8:30 and lasted only a few minutes. This meeting, in the same conference room as the one just fourteen hours earlier, was not nearly as emotional. It was no secret that some of the other managers had been saying bad things about me lately—that I was becoming lazy and was not pulling my load. Some of those in the meeting were great friends, but many of them were just as happy to see me go; such is the reality of bearing the CFS label. After a few handshakes and a roomful of goodbyes, the meeting was quickly adjourned.

As I walked back to my office, I noticed that there was already a memo on the bulletin board announcing my departure. There are few long goodbyes in broadcasting.

I took my pictures and awards down from the walls and packed them into boxes Hettie had collected for me the night before. I gathered some videotapes and a few other possessions, loaded up some personal files and destroyed some others, and carried the load out to the parking lot and my waiting car. The last thing I did before turning in my keys was remove the *Tim Kenny, News Director* sign from my office door. That person ceased to exist at 9:50 A.M. on August 21, 1991. Nearly two years after Hurricane Hugo, I was again dust in the wind.

13

UNEMPLOYMENT "COMPENSATION"

The first few days after leaving my job were each a challenge to endure.

I had made myself a few promises that morning when I packed my belongings and left WPDE. I wasn't going to become a bum. No soap operas or game shows, no sitting around in pajamas, no unshaven face day after day. I would keep a schedule and be up and dressed every morning, trying as best I could to remain productive.

Surely my old colleagues would call frequently needing help with this problem or that, I told myself. Surely I would remain a viable member of the media and of the local business community. I couldn't just go from taking calls from the governor and senators to being nothing at all, overnight. Surely it didn't work that way.

Surely, I was as wrong as I could be.

My former colleagues didn't call, even though the news department remained a ship without a captain for several months after I left. I later found that management had posted a note instructing them not to call, which I still do not understand. I still had a mind, I still had ideas, I could still solve problems. Why wasn't anyone interested? Was it perhaps that I was easier to deal with now that my confusing illness and its strange name and weird symptoms were were completely out of sight? Was Tim Kenny just too much trouble?

I spent my first few days of unemployment doing odd jobs around the house. The first day I replaced or adjusted all of the magnets on the kitchen cabinet doors. The second day I fixed some other damaged hardware. By the third day, I was out of projects to keep my mind off my situation. I sat in silence and stared out the front door.

I returned to Dr. Cheney's office that Friday for my infusion. Sheryl Autry asked me how I was adjusting to my new life.

"Fine," I said simply.

It was on that first drive back from Charlotte after leaving my career that I noticed the long empty stretch of highway leading up to the narrow concrete bridge. The opportunity seemed perfect.

There was no traffic in either direction. I shoved the accelerator down and watched my tachometer climb toward the red zone. Seventy miles per hour—then eighty. The steering wheel began to feel light in my hands as the narrow bridge loomed closer and closer.

The speedometer needle passed ninety, then one hundred. I was almost to the bridge. Then—105 miles per hour. I knew any loss of control at this speed would be fatal.

Suddenly a truck appeared, coming toward me. I stood on the brake, my car rocking back and forth as I pulled in the reins and dropped back to the speed limit.

I might be trying to kill myself, but I wouldn't hurt someone else in the process.

I really had no active desire to end my life. I had access to guns and strong drugs that would have made the process foolproof, had that been my intention. Instead I wanted to tempt fate to see if it would take me out of this horrible existence. If the fates had cast this lot in my life, perhaps they would provide me a fitting exit, as well.

Dr. Robertson probed that part of my thinking on my next visit.

"Have you spent much time rethinking the value of your life?" he asked.

That was about all I'd done in the past week. Dr. Robertson asked what I planned on doing about that feeling.

"If you mean, 'Am I going to kill myself?' the answer is no," I told him. "But if you mean, 'Do I wish I were dead?' the answer is yes."

"Why?"

"Why? Because I have no life," I said. "It's over. And I hate sitting around and waiting for . . ."

"For what?"

"For *it* to happen!" I said. "The sentence has already been handed down. Why wait to have it carried out?"

I looked across the desk at Robertson, knowing what his job was in that situation, knowing what he must be thinking, knowing what he would try to say. I honestly felt bad for him. Despite being in my own private hell, I felt bad that I was making life difficult for another person.

"Look," I explained, "you don't have to try to do this. I know what's happening here, and I'm not going to change it. I'm not going to become a happy sick person—there is nothing in the world you can do or say to make that happen. Nothing. I've read the stories about the quadriplegic who paints by holding the brush in her teeth, and I admire her. But I'm not going to become like that. My life is over, plain and simple."

But Dr. Robertson hit to the core of my thinking with his next statement. "You don't have a job, so you're not worth anything—is that what you think? You might as well be dead, is that it? You're not actually going to kill yourself, but if something bad just happened, that would be okay, right?"

Bingo! I respected this guy. He really knew where I was coming from. I told him about the narrow bridge.

"That's you . . . that's Tim Kenny," he said. "Just sitting around trying to get well isn't for him. He's got to be in the thick of things, solving everyone's problems, carrying everyone's burdens . . . and if he can't have that, he'd rather go out in a blaze of glory on some country road somewhere."

That's exactly how I felt, and I wasn't about to let Dr. Robertson or anyone else change my mind. Still, I knew he'd try. That's what I was paying him for.

"How long have you been working this hard?" Dr. Robertson asked, making some notes in a way that was starting to get on my nerves.

I'd been working full-time since I was fourteen years old, I told him as if I were dictating his notes for him. I spent summers and nights on the job during my school years, working as many as three jobs at other times. I had actually left college because it bored me. There was more to the world than listening to people teach. I could learn by doing. I could change the world by doing. I couldn't change anything by sitting around. Dr. Robertson continued to take notes as I gave a brief history of my working life. When I felt I needed to, I paused in my monologue to allow him to catch up with his notes. He'd look up and I'd continue.

"What about your adolescence?" he asked. "What do you remember of that?"

Here it comes, I thought. Time to heal the inner child and make me a well-adjusted adult—the psychobabble of the 1990s! I might listen to everything else he had to say, but I wasn't going to play into this nonsense.

"Everything was *fine*," I answered.

Robertson kept pushing. Finally, I decided to give him the truth. He was a likable person, and I had promised him in our first meeting that I would never lie.

I didn't really have much of an adolescence, I admitted. I went to school and I worked. I was married by the time I was twenty. All of my life had been work. That was my identity.

"You see, that's part of your problem in dealing with this," Dr. Robertson insisted. "This would be a terrible blow to anyone, but most people have a core identity to fall back on. For you, that identity is working hard, helping people, achieving goals. Take that away and you have nothing."

I squirmed in the chair for the first time since I'd met this guy. As a reflex I glanced at my watch.

"Look at the time," I said sarcastically, as if I had somewhere to be. "Time for me to go. I'm sure you have a client waiting."

"Next week?" Dr. Robertson asked, making a few more notes.

"Sure, what the heck," I said. "I'll stop and make another appointment on my way out."

He walked me to the door and we shook hands.

Sixty minutes later, I was speeding toward the concrete bridge.

* * *

I had wrapped myself so tightly in denial during my final few months on the job that I really had no idea just how sick I had become. In the weeks immediately following my departure from WPDE, my illness—so obvious to others—became more and more apparent to me.

I still maintained my schedule of getting up and dressed every day. I still refused to watch daytime TV. But I no longer had the strength to complete the list of household tasks I made. There were no more trips to the hardware store, no more tinkering with this or that to wile the hours away.

I couldn't drive to Myrtle Beach to see my friends. I couldn't go to lunch or dinner with Hettie. I couldn't walk around the block or even down the street. And thanks to my scattered brain, I could hardly read. I had several books I wanted to complete, but the words just danced around the pages.

A few weeks later, Dr. Cheney and I spent about thirty minutes talking in an exam room. I was feeling worse, and my left eyelid was drooping. My thinking was again clouded and slow, and I often had a difficult time finishing my sentences.

Cheney attributed the problems to continuing brain injury, a condition that is covered very generally by the term *encephalopathy*. He had long held the belief that a virus was a major part of CFS, and in my case (because of my concussion) and many other cases, the virus had made its way into the brain. The drooping eye, he explained, could be caused by a swelling in the brain pressing on one of two nerves in the area. The other problems were typical in my type of CFS.

The drooping eye was the first visible reminder for me that I was not well, and I didn't appreciate it one bit. If I sat straight up in a chair and the lighting didn't reveal the circles under my eyes, I generally looked the same as I had when I was healthy. Because I couldn't exercise and my metabolism was operating at about sixty percent of normal, I had gained a few pounds, but a stranger wouldn't know that. My drooping eye, however, was a giveaway that something was wrong.

When I mentioned the problem to Dr. Robertson, he made some notes and he got me to admit that I was lucky I could see.

The eye problem might be temporary, he said, but it was far from terrible.

Dr. Cheney wanted to measure my brain injury as best he could using a relatively new test called brain topography—a sort of map of the brain. Whereas a CAT scan or an MRI forms architectural models of the brain (actual pictures of its structure and flaws), the brain map forms a functional model of the brain. To the skilled interpreter, it shows what parts of the brain are working and how well under varying circumstances.

A few days after the test Dr. Cheney had the results.

"Let's say you didn't know anything about me," I said. "You see this test—what do you conclude?"

Cheney was thoughtful for a moment, studying the various computer-generated pictures from the brain map. He wanted to answer my question honestly.

"Well, there are some possible explanations," he began, still studying the images. "You could be suffering from severely advanced multiple sclerosis . . . maybe your liver's gone south and it's pumping ammonia into your brain, wiping it out . . . those are two possible explanations."

"Anything else?" I asked.

"Well, more than anything," he said, "if I saw this test and didn't know anything about you, I'd look at the fact that your sleep wave is dominant; that you have very little alpha wave at all. I'd see these areas here," he said, pointing to dark spots on the pictures, "and I'd see that those parts of your brain are working at very low levels. All in all, I think I'd say you'd been beaten over the head with a baseball bat and were about to go into a coma. Of course, I know your medical history, and you have no history of being beaten over the head with a baseball bat."

Dr. Cheney smiled.

The brain map confirmed that as my body became capable of less and less, my brain was following suit—or perhaps even leading the way.

It wasn't enough that I was sick. I was becoming stupid, too. For the first time since I'd become ill, I began to feel hopeless about the future. My attitude wasn't lost on Hettie. She tried to talk me into doing whatever I could to pass the time, maybe buying a computer and learning something new. "You've always wanted to write," she said. "Now's your chance."

She was right. I'd always wanted to be a writer, but writing now—under these circumstances—would be therapy, not a career. I wasn't going to learn to paint with my teeth. I wasn't going to become a well-adjusted sick person. I was mad as hell, and nobody was going to change that.

But with Hettie's urging, I eventually bought the computer and began to make plans for writing the Great American Novel; this would be a career, not therapy, I vowed. *Everybody* tries to write the Great American Novel, even people who've been hit over the head with a baseball bat.

Dr. Robertson also worked to turn the tide on my sagging spirits, but I refused to respond to him. I met with him each week, but I still sped toward the concrete bridge hoping I'd blow a tire or something. He later told me—in an admission that frightens me now—that every time we'd say goodbye, he realized it might be the last time we'd meet. I was, he admitted, trying hard to let my imagined death sentence come to pass.

Dr. Robertson's main area of attack was my contention that my work was my life, and that without it I had nothing. What about Hettie, he'd always ask. What about the people whose careers I'd helped? Didn't they make life worth living?

As far as Hettie was concerned, I felt as if I were already a dismal failure as a husband and getting worse by the minute. As far as people whose careers I'd helped, they were getting along fine without me. Sure, when WPDE hired a new news director, everybody told me he was nothing like I'd been. But somehow the world continued to turn without me. The newscasts weren't as good as they once were (the ratings confirmed that), but they still got on the air everyday. I used to think that simple feat would be impossible without me there.

CFS teaches you—if nothing else—that none of us is irreplaceable.

Then one day Dr. Robertson told me a story that made a serious impression. He told me about certain religions that do not focus on an afterlife, and how people within those faiths leave behind memorials such as hospital wings and scholarship funds to keep their memories alive.

"Think of your accomplishments in that way," he urged me. "The ratings you achieved, the careers you started, the people you helped . . . they're all living memorials to your accomplishments. You don't have to be dead for your successes to matter—they matter right now. Wherever these people go in their careers, they'll be taking a part of you with them. They couldn't be where they are today without you—*their* success is *your* success!"

I had to admit that Dr. Robertson's thinking made sense—at least he was making sense for someone who might be trying to become a well-adjusted sick person. But since I had no such intentions, I was merely intrigued by his story. I quickly filed it away. The desire to live still eluded me, and I still existed in a very dangerous place. I kept speeding toward that concrete bridge.

Six months into my forced retirement, my brother offered to take me on a plane ride. Bob had recently earned his own pilot's license, and he was eager to take his younger brother flying. I hadn't been in a plane in over a year, so I jumped at his offer.

"Where to?" Bob asked.

I thought about my friend Tom Sorrells, now a weathercaster in Columbus, Ohio. I always disliked just flying around town, burning up the sky, as I called it. There was nothing like taking off from one place and landing somewhere else. *That* was flying!

"Columbus," I told Bob. "But first let me call Tommy."

Tom met us at the Ohio State University Airport, and within five seconds, I knew this trip was the best therapy I could have asked for. I was still feeling self-conscious about the extra weight I had gained, my pale appearance, and my drooping eyelid, and I was wondering what tales Tommy had heard about my departure from WPDE from people who did not understand. But Tom's huge bear hug made all of that disappear.

"Where to, Bubba?" he asked. I hadn't been called "Bubba" since Tommy had left South Carolina nine months earlier.

I told him I wanted to see his apartment and then his television station. I wanted to meet his boss, tour his newsroom, and stand in the exact spot where he did his weathercasts. I also wanted to tour the competing station where Mitra—Tommy's girlfriend and another of my former employees—worked as assignment editor and producer.

Our visit to Columbus lasted just over three hours, but I got to see all that I had come for. Standing in Tommy's weather spot, I pictured him on the air in the sixteenth-largest city in America. I also imagined once again being his backup or his boss, and we traded war stories about some of our old TV adventures. I was never more proud of my friend and this young man whose career I had impacted. We posed for a treasured photograph on his anchor desk.

At Mitra's station, I was buoyed by her accomplishments as well. I had hired her immediately after college, made her a reporter, and given her a chance to taste newsroom management. Now Mitra was using those talents at a huge state-of-the-art television station, quite an accomplishment for a twenty-four-year-old.

As we walked into the parking lot, her station's news helicopter clawed its way into the Columbus sky only a few hundred yards from where we stood. I reminded Mitra of one of her first assignments in South Carolina—a firemen's appreciation banquet on a rainy night where she'd been both reporter and photographer. Her weekly salary then was probably less than an hour's flying time cost in the helicopter she'd just dispatched. How far she'd come, and how proud it made me feel.

Bob flew me back to Pennsylvania, and a day later I returned to South Carolina. Nothing in my life had actually changed in those few days, but I was finally beginning to see Dr. Robertson's point about my accomplishments living on through other people. It certainly wasn't as satisfying as doing the impossible myself, but this new feeling lifted my spirits enough that I began to be thankful for the life I had lived, and I began to wonder about what I might accomplish in the future.

I thought of one of my favorite old movies, *The Flight of the Phoenix*, starring another western Pennsylvanian, Jimmy Stewart.

In the movie, a giant airplane crashes in the desert. The survivors use the pieces of the useless airplane to build a smaller craft they hope will fly them to safety. Some of the survivors doubt the project will work, but most of them go along with the effort. After all, there was little else to do but wait to die, and there was always the chance that the crazy scheme would work.

I considered using the movie as a working model for my own life. I had certainly been strong and capable when I crashed, and I was now lost in the desert. But maybe I could rebuild my life in some small way, maybe as a writer, maybe in some other capacity.

In Greek mythology, the Phoenix is a giant bird that lives for five hundred years in great splendor and beauty. At the end of its life, the Phoenix builds its own funeral pyre to be totally consumed in the blaze. From the fire's ashes, the legend says, a new Phoenix arises.

It was a metaphor that intrigued me more and more as I considered it. It didn't instantly turn me into the well-adjusted sick person I vowed I'd never become, but seeing that my legacy was alive and well in others had given me more hope than I'd had in a year. I had always welcomed challenges in the past, and the one that lay before me now was greater than any I had ever faced before.

Could I make a new life from the ashes of the old? Could I still make a difference in the world? Or was this all some coping mechanism that would pass in a few days, only to leave me empty and depressed, left to wander the desert until I died?

I didn't know the answer immediately, and I still had many more battles to fight. But I do know that I started to drive more carefully, and I was no longer speeding toward that concrete bridge.

14

THE DISABILITY WARS

"Brain mapping shows significant delta wave formation with a virtual absence of beta and alpha. Delta wave predominance is indicative of brain injury . . . [and] correlates with Tim's severe neurocognitive symptomatology. . . .

"Tim's objective findings correlate with the severity of his severe constitutional and neurocognitive symptoms and I strongly feel he is totally disabled from any employment in the national economy, even the most sedentary, part-time position. . . ."

—Paul R. Cheney, M.D., February 24, 1992, in a disability letter
written on behalf of the author

My ex-employer, Diversified Communications, was supportive and helpful during my illness and the period after my disability. But even Diversified has limits; it is, after all, a business, and not a social welfare organization.

Under the terms of my company's benefits policy, I was to receive full pay and benefits for 180 days after my illness forced me out of my position. This is an extremely considerate policy and most CFS patients are not as lucky as I to have had such a great company behind them.

Wherever I go and meet with CFS patients, I almost universally hear horror stories about their disability insurance process. One executive, who was stricken with CFS before the disease even had a name, left his job still undiagnosed and walked away from hundreds of thousands of dollars in potential disability insurance payments.

I know of others whose employers had no disability insurance policy whatsoever, and still others who were self-employed and had no corporate support. There are others who may have been covered by some sort of disability policy, but the policy's underwriters refused to recognize CFS as a legitimate illness. And Social Security—well, I'll get to that later.

My benefit period was to end at midnight February 15, 1992. At that moment Diversified Communications would terminate me—the "T word," Liz had called it—and I would be officially without a job for the first time since high school. Of course, I hadn't worked a single day in that six months, but I was still technically an employee, and that meant something to me. When February 15 passed, even that designation would be taken away.

I watched the calendar closely as 1991 came to an end and 1992 began, dreading the approach of the "T word."

There was nothing special about February 15. There were no calls, no letters, no papers to sign. What would happen at midnight that night would be automatic. It had been decided six months earlier. All I could do was let it happen.

I am not one to let any occasion pass without making note of it—perhaps that is why I choose to write. And so as the sun set on February 15 and my tenure with Diversified Communications drew to an official close, I considered how I might spend my final hours on the payroll.

By eleven o'clock Hettie was asleep beside me, and I stared in the darkness toward the digital clock on the other side of our bedroom. For nearly twenty minutes, my thoughts followed no particular pattern, except that I was getting more depressed with each change on the clock. The sense of regret and dread that had been present earlier in the day were worsening as the minutes passed, and I felt the lonely world becoming colder by the second.

At 11:22, I finally came up with a more constructive plan.

Rather than lie in bed and feel sorry for myself about what I'd lost, I would spend the time between then and midnight reliving the wonderful highlights of a tremendous career.

I thought of Hurricane Hugo, and how much my planning had done to make our station's coverage a success. I thought of the first time I had ever seen a President in person; the first time I ever picked up the phone to find it was the governor. I remembered flying with the Thunderbirds twice, slipping the bonds of gravity and playing in the tall clouds from the cockpit of the $20-million F-16. I remembered meeting stars in Los Angeles, slipping off to a baseball game at Dodger Stadium, jetting across the country with someone else paying the bill.

I thought of the young people whose careers I had started or shaped. I thought of the people I'd hired who had found mates after coming to work for me—an awesome feeling. (To date, my hiring has resulted in three marriages.) I remembered hard news stories, light stories, and stories of great sadness. There were investigative reports that made headlines and silly reports that made people laugh. I recalled the days of being a smiling weathercaster, of going into schools and speaking to kids, of always making the time to talk with someone interested in a career in broadcasting.

I relived the moment more than a decade earlier when I had knocked on the door at WPDE looking for work and knowing nothing about television.

I recalled staff meetings and strategy sessions, awards banquets and parades, logos on tee shirts and decals on news cars. I tried to remember it all that night and I think that I did.

And then the clock changed from 11:59 to 12:00. I was now officially unemployed. I took one final look at the clock, rolled over, and went to sleep.

When I woke up the next morning, I had one more worry to confront: paying the bills.

I had always felt young and invincible and had never even considered disability insurance before I became ill. Fortunately, Diversified Communications had included it in its benefit package for most employees, and as my 180 days wore on, I began to learn all I could about it.

While laws vary from state to state, most insurance policies allow employees disabled from non-work-related illnesses to collect only a certain percentage of their previous salary. The idea behind this, I've been told, is not to make disability a profitable experience. Fat chance.

In South Carolina at the time, the law allowed insurers to pay a disabled worker no more than sixty percent of his or her pre-disability salary. I knew that would be a major pay cut, but I thought Social Security would step in and pick up the balance, or at least get me close to my earlier income level. Hettie and I did not live high, but like most young couples, we needed every penny we earned.

We had a small home—our first—and a healthy mortgage payment. Hettie was an itinerant teacher, traveling up to a hundred miles a day, so she needed a full-size automobile. (South Carolina has one of the highest highway death rates in the nation; I was never comfortable with her driving so much.) I also needed a car, even though I didn't work, because of my trips to Charlotte. We had student loans, a significant tax liability as a two-income, no-children family, and other miscellaneous debts. And we were working hard to get Hettie through a Master's program at an expensive college in upstate South Carolina. Looking at all of that, I didn't see anywhere to cut expenses by forty percent.

I had begun the disability insurance claims process long before February 16, hoping to have everything handled in plenty of time before that date. Unfortunately, just a few days before the insurance company was to begin paying me, the company called with dreadful news: It wouldn't approve my claim. It needed more time to evaluate my case.

I was furious. I had sent the company every bit of medical information I had accumulated since my first symptoms had appeared. It had the results from every test, every office visit, every evaluation. As an Ampligen patient, I'd been put through an extensive battery of additional tests that only strengthened the case that I was disabled—the CDC and FDA had agreed I represented an extreme CFS case—but the insurance company still balked. If the CDC and FDA agreed that I was sick, what was the problem?

At first I was told the problem was that I had "too much documentation." How can you have too much documentation of anything? I wondered. The more I called and the angrier I got, the less responsive the company became. February 16 came and went and my claim was still officially "under review." Considering house payments and car loans, I prayed this impasse wouldn't last long. Still, the insurance company offered no hope of when—or even *if*—my claim might be approved.

Then came word that I would need something called an IME—an independent medical exam. I would have to see a doctor chosen by the insurance company to screen people who'd applied for disability benefits. "Okay," I told the claims representative, "let me fax you a list of CFS specialists around the world. You pick the one I should see."

But it didn't work that way; the company didn't want me to see a CFS specialist. It wanted me to see one of its doctors. This sent me into another angry dissertation.

CFS is still an emerging illness, largely misunderstood and undiagnosed, I told them. "You can't just send me to any doctor and expect him to understand my case," I pleaded.

But the claims representative said that under the terms of the policy that's exactly what it could do.

I'll never forget the claims representative's words when I mentioned Dr. Cheney and his credentials as the world's top CFS clinician: "We *know* what he's all about," she said. "We know what Dr. Cheney represents. We want *another* opinion."

I continued to argue this point for a few more days, and got nowhere. I would have to play by the company's rules. I called the claims representative and asked her to please rush the IME. I had bills to pay. She countered that there was no way to rush the appointment, that it could take several weeks to set up and evaluate.

This infuriated me, but I stayed calm on the phone. I would be nice and I would remain cooperative, I'd promised myself.

There was simply no other way to go. My financial survival was at stake.

And then, out of the blue, my claims representative made this strange comment: "Our doctor thinks it's unusual that you haven't been examined by a psychologist. Why hasn't anyone suggested the MMPI test?"

This again! If I'd simply been disabled on the basis of clinical depression, my claim would have been settled weeks ago. But since my doctor maintained I had a physiological illness, I had gummed up the works and made everyone suspicious.

"I have taken the MMPI," I told her, and filled her in on my visits with Dr. Robertson (which had ended about a month earlier).

That changed everything.

"Get us those records as soon as you can," the claims representative said. "Maybe we can clear this up after all."

In the meantime the company issued me a "conditional" check for my first month's benefit. It was money, but I really didn't consider it mine. If the company ultimately refused my claim, I'd have to repay it. I was thankful for the cash flow, but I was beginning to feel overwhelmed by the stress of fighting yet another battle.

It was at about that time, after another long and frustrating conversation with the insurance company, that I quite seriously considering just giving up. I had been abused by doctors, pharmacists, co-workers, strangers, friends, friends' doctors—and now this. I remember hanging up the telephone, slumping forward with my face in my hands, and thinking that I'd just plain had enough. "There's just no fight left in me," I told Hettie. That night was the closest I'd come to suicide in my entire CFS experience. I felt that I'd finally been beaten.

But in the coming days I bounced back, and I rushed Dr. Robertson's office along to release my records. I was concerned about how I'd scored on the MMPI, especially since I'd heard a lecture about the peculiar scores of CFS patients. Dr. Robertson told me not to worry; my scores were consistent with the "chronic pain" curve on the MMPI profile. I absolutely hated the thought that my insurance claim boiled down to how I'd performed on one simple test—I always hated being put into categories.

Dr. Robertson was training a new secretary, so typing up my results took longer than I'd expected, adding even more stress. Finally, after several days, I got the word I'd been waiting for: the records had been mailed. Now I had to once again wait for some doctor in another state to review may case.

A few days later, the call came: my claim had been officially approved. The stress mill had halted, at least for a while.

Receiving only sixty percent of your previous salary can be a pretty attractive scenario if the alternative is receiving nothing. It wasn't really sixty percent, because I now had to pay for my own health and life insurance (previously job benefits). So I was making almost half of what I had before. But considering all I had been through with the disability insurance company, that half was much appreciated. Now, I reasoned, a few weeks of dealing with Social Security and I would be financially back on track.

Not exactly.

My insurance company promptly asked me to begin the Social Security process, and it informed me that whatever amount I received from Social Security would be deducted from its monthly checks. No matter how much I got from my government disability benefits, I would still receive only that sixty percent of my previous salary. I was totally flabbergasted.

"Read your policy," the claims representative said.

But after my initial disappointment and wondering again how I would make ends meet, I finally began the lengthy process of applying for my Social Security benefits. I had paid into the program for nearly twenty years; it seemed only right that it would pick up a portion of my disability tab.

I'd heard that virtually everyone is turned down the first time he or she applies for Social Security disability payments, and that's exactly what happened to me. So, only days after the initial denial (a mere formality, I'd heard), I filed an application to have my case reviewed.

All of my records went to the South Carolina Disability Determination Office for the formal review. The state office ordered another evaluation with Dr. Cheney, paying him a whopping twenty-five dollars for his time. The office sent me piles of paperwork asking questions about how well I could kneel or crawl and whether I could stand up very long. I wrote several pages of notes about my job history, going back to the days of spending summers in a sheet metal shop or as a greenskeeper. Somehow I failed to understand what raking sand traps on a golf course had to do with my ability to be a news director, but I knew that my only chance with the government was to respond to its every request.

Another two months passed before I heard from the Social Security Administration. Its response was priceless:

> You do have some limitations in your ability to work. You can stand and/or walk with normal breaks for a total of at least two hours in an eight-hour workday. You can sit with normal breaks for a total of about six hours in an eight-hour workday. . . . You can occasionally climb or balance, stoop or kneel, crouch or crawl. In your description of your past job as a TV news/promotion director you said that you had occasionally lifted over 100 pounds, and frequently lifted up to 25 pounds with occasional bending, and walked or stood up to eight hours a day. However, as it is described in the national economy, this job requires lifting 10 pounds maximum, walking or standing only occasionally up to two hours a day. Based on the way this job is performed in the national economy, we have concluded that you can return to your past job as a TV news and promotion director.

Thus, in the considered opinion of the Social Security Administration, I was fine. It had sagely concluded that I could do my old job, no questions asked. This was the bureaucratic crowning jewel to the miserable experience I'd endured for more than three years. Were it not so incredibly important for my long-term finances, the letter would have made me laugh for the first time in months!

I read the climactic sentence again and again: "we have concluded that you can return to your past job . . ." That was incredible! I couldn't even *read* a newspaper, let alone run a news depart-

ment! But according to the Social Security Administration, I was
healed! All I needed to do now was place an ad in *Broadcasting*
magazine:

> *Television News Director.* Unable to work Mondays or
> Fridays because of experimental drug therapy, without
> which I might end up in the hospital. Other days, may be
> able to arrive at work by 5:00 or 6:00 P.M., provided I am
> able to shower and dress. Occasionally able to climb or bal-
> ance, stoop or kneel, crouch or crawl. Must have lied on
> my Social Security disability application about sixteen-
> hour days, seven-day weeks, and heavy lifting of cable
> spools, editing machines, and other equipment. Highly
> dyslexic especially after fatigue. Unable to make decisions
> or find words quickly, and am subject to extreme memory
> failures. Highly sensitive to intense light. Current IQ is
> approximately forty points lower than when last held news
> position. Can neither walk around the block nor balance a
> checkbook, but have experience with a million-dollar
> operating budget and highly technical designs and installa-
> tions.

I can hear my phone ringing off the hook now.

Fortunately, Social Security's denial had no immediate impact
on my finances, since my private disability insurance payments
would have been reduced by the amount of my award anyway. But
this determination had long-term consequences.

Eventually, I presumed, my disability insurance company would
tire of paying me on a claim labeled "chronic fatigue syndrome."
When that day came, Social Security payments would be the difference between Hettie and I and financial disaster. I prayed each
month that the insurance company would continue to view my
claim as the legitimate matter that it was, and I offered a prayer of
thanks when every check came.

Also—though I don't completely understand the law—I would
soon be unable to maintain my health insurance through my former employer's group policy. It was highly unlikely that I would be

able to obtain private health coverage. Many insurance companies will not pay CFS medical claims because they say the disease is not a "real" illness. Those same companies, however, will not sell health or life insurance to CFS patients because they say the disease is a preexisting and potentially life-threatening condition. Thus, a Social Security determination of disability would mean that at least I'd have Medicare to fall back on.

There is one more thing about Social Security's denial that bothers me: For many patients, it is the only option. They have no private insurance, as I did. The delays I endured and the final determination I received would be a financial death knell to thousands of patients. I've met many of them—real people who have lost their homes, their cars, everything they've worked their entire lives to accumulate. I'm not talking about people who can't afford HBO and Cinemax; I'm talking about people who are a hair's breadth from being out on the street.

As I considered the ticking clock of my private disability insurance and wondered how much longer I could buy my former company's health and life insurance, there remained only one solution I could imagine for this entire mess. I had to get well again; I had to reenter the work force somehow.

I didn't know how or when that would happen, but as I would sit up nights looking at the walls around me and hearing the hum of the refrigerator from down the hall, I knew that there seemed to be simply no other option. Our house, the food in the refrigerator, everything we owned, seemed to depend on me getting back to work someday. And I used to think the pressure of the television business was immense!

Two final points about the topic of disability insurance: First, there is an incredible irony to the entire Social Security process. I had paid into that fund since I was fourteen, because that was the law. Then, when I needed it most, the government turned down my request for benefits, based apparently upon my ability to kneel and crawl. The moment I would return to work, however, you can be sure of one thing: Social Security tax would be collected before I even saw my first paycheck.

Second—speaking for myself and every other CFS patient I have met who has undergone the miserable process of disability insurance claims and financial disaster—*we don't want to have to take one penny of the insurance money!* We don't want to have to rely on private insurance or Social Security. We only want one thing: to be well again. Then we can go back to work, back to making a living, back to providing for our families, back to contributing to the economy, back to saving for the future.

But until that happens, we still have to pay the bills.

15

THE "F WORD"

The middle of a television interview is no time to get emotional, but I just couldn't hold back my feelings.

I was sitting in my home with the chief medical correspondent from CNN trying to act composed and informed, trying to put forth the best image I could under the circumstances. But his question caught me off guard, and my reaction leapt out.

He asked if I'd had any kind of psychiatric history—any mental illness. The question seemed to come out of nowhere; we'd been discussing the realities of CFS and what it had done to a formerly productive television news manager.

In a matter of seconds, every emotion of the past few years passed through my mind. I was hurt, angry, disappointed, even furious that he asked that question. The last emotion to cross my mind was sadness, because more than anything else I am saddened that so many people still think CFS patients are crazy.

I tried to blink away what felt like tears starting in the corners of my eyes. I hadn't expected him to ask if I had a mental disorder. He had been studying CFS; he had to know otherwise. I was sane and I was sick—he knew that coming into the interview. Then why the sucker-punch?

It was too late. The low *whirrrr* of the camera's zoom lens told me that this moment would make it on the air. Here was an extreme close-up of a CFS patient misty-eyed, another point for people who doubt the disease exists. This was the exact opposite of the image I'd wanted to portray, but the question cut right to the core of a very painful issue.

Noting my instant reaction, the interviewer asked me a follow-up question: "Do you think that's a fair question?"

"Maybe it's a fair question," I said, "but ask yourself this: Would you ask that question to someone with diabetes, cancer, AIDS? Why only CFS? Why do people only ask *us* about mental illness?"

I knew the answer already. It was the same reason I'd been misunderstood by friends and co-workers since I was first diagnosed, it was the same reason I had such a hard time with my disability insurance claim, the same reason I was turned down for Social Security benefits.

It was the "F word." *Fatigue.*

People close to this illness, those who research or treat it, those who fight for congressional funding on Capitol Hill, those who lead support groups or write newsletters, have all become accustomed to the name chronic fatigue syndrome. But the public has not. To them, the name trivializes this disorder. As one friend told me recently how someone had asked about my condition: "Isn't that the thing where you fall asleep all the time?"

Simply put, I've come to learn that the "F word" is the single greatest obstacle to understanding, research, diagnosis, and treatment of this illness. In a world consumed with AIDS, heart disease, breast implant dangers, and the harmful effects of secondhand smoke, few people have time for a group of patients who bear the brand of the "F word."

Frankly, I don't blame them.

I've seen studies that indicate as much as twenty percent of the population claim to be fatigued an unusual amount of the time. Many of them even consider themselves to be "chronically fatigued," and I'm sure they are: life in the 1990s can do that to you. But these people do not have the disease I have written about in this book, they do not have the disease that has shattered families, destroyed careers, taken lives, and ripped through entire communities like a vicious tornado. They are tired, but rest and better living habits will help them.

Unfortunately, considering the name of our illness, most people think the same about us: Get some sleep, take a few weeks

and everything will be okay. Or, as in the case of the TV interviewer, people look for an explanation in one of the greatest causes
of fatigue—depression.

I do not mean to trivialize depression, for it is an extremely
serious clinical and psychological illness. But depression is not
what we have. We have a serious disorder that disrupts the
immune system, degenerates muscle tissue, destroys normal metabolism, robs our memory and thinking abilities, and causes severe
brain damage, among other things. This is real—it is not imagined.
It does not begin in our minds.

Unfortunately, in today's busy society, a name is everything.
"Chronic fatigue syndrome" translates into "being tired a lot."

I've mentioned before that there are many more female than
male CFS patients, though the reasons for that are unclear. I think
those demographics have played an insidious role in slowing the
realization that this disease is serious. Women are just not taken as
seriously as men by the medical profession. For years doctors have
been seeing women complaining of terrible weakness, pain, and a
list of other symptoms that fit no known pattern, and many of
those doctors have dismissed the women's complaints.

"Get some rest."

"Find a hobby."

"Get a job outside the home."

These are hardly notions that dig deeply for the truth at the
heart of this strange malady.

I find it poetic justice that two of the most well-known pio-
neers in CFS research are females: Dr. Elaine DeFreitis, formerly of
the Wistar Institute in Pennsylvania, and Dr. Nancy Klimas of the
University of Miami. DeFreitis was one of the first to find retrovi-
ral sequences in CFS patients. Klimas was one of the first to document the severe immunological abnormalities among the CFS
patient population. Women—and men—everywhere owe them a
great debt of gratitude. But as long as the name of this illness they
continue to investigate bears the "F word," there will be no great
outpouring of support for their work, despite the fact that current
figures suggest CFS is already at epidemic levels—far more common than multiple sclerosis, for example, and possibly as serious.

mon than multiple sclerosis, for example, and possibly as serious. Some research even implies that CFS may be caused by a new retrovirus—the same nasty family of virus that causes AIDS. More startling is the fact that this same research cannot find CFS risk groups; we could be seeing a *casually transmitted* retrovirus, one of the most serious health threats of our time. But as long as the "F word" persists, few people other than the patients themselves and a handful of dedicated researchers will care.

I see examples everyday of how people do not take this illness seriously—even people who should know better. Not long after a full-page article appeared in my local paper about my sickness and how it had ended my career and taken almost everything else away, I was talking to a travel agent I know.

"Sorry to read about you in the paper," he said. "It's just all that stress you were under, man. Get some rest . . . you'll be fine."

Then a well-intentioned neighbor invited me to an outdoor sporting event at a time when I didn't even have the ability to walk down my own driveway.

"Getting out in the sun will help. Being around people will make you feel better," he said kindly.

If being around people could help my condition, I'd camp out at Madison Square Garden. If rest could cure me, I'd study how to become Rip Van Winkle.

But I really don't blame these people for jumping to faulty conclusions. They are reacting to the "F word." With a disease where the patients often look healthy, fatigue sounds like a simple problem to overcome. I have often said it would be easier for people to understand my limitations if I were in a body cast, or if I—like many CFS patients—needed a cane to get around on.

But there is a simpler way to bring about public and medical understanding of this disease: Change the name!

The Centers for Disease Control established the name and diagnostic criteria for chronic fatigue syndrome in 1988. We have since learned enough about this disease to fill a medical library! Why does the name persist?

It is a complex and speculative issue, and people close to

ment conspiracy around every corner, here is what I think is happening.

First, the CDC was reluctant to even admit there was such an illness back in the mid-1980s when Drs. Cheney and Peterson called them to Nevada. CDC was up to its initials in another major problem it had dropped the ball on—AIDS—and it surely didn't need a new disease to concern itself with. Maybe—as I believe some bureaucrats had tried with AIDS—if it just ignored this thing, these people would snap out of it. After all, several public health agencies at one time informally referred to AIDS as "gay cancer"—quite an impotent and unfeeling reaction from the government organizations charged with protecting public health.

Another government agency, the National Institutes of Health—one notch above CDC in the bureaucratic pecking order—also shares the blame. NIH has long held that CFS isn't real. Even though many of its top researchers are now convinced that this is a serious disease, a government agency cannot simply reverse position easily.

Don't believe me? How long did it take us to get out of Vietnam even after we knew we couldn't win? That will be the subject of debate for decades. Yes, politicians and political appointees will sacrifice lives to save face. They have done it before, and they will do it again.

I am told that the government says it will change the chronic fatigue syndrome name whenever a causative agent is found. History hardly supports that position (and the current level of government research funding will hardly help find the agent). Consider a few conditions named *before* the cause was found: Legionnaire's Disease, toxic shock syndrome, cystic fibrosis, multiple sclerosis. (Incredibly, the last was initially thought to be a strange form of mental illness!) You could find dozens more in a medical encyclopedia. We don't know what causes lymphoma, a serious form of cancer, but we sure don't call it "Bump Under the Arm Syndrome." Twentieth-century medical history simply does not contain examples of serious illnesses being benignly named after a single symptom. If it happened that way, as Dr. Cheney once told an interviewer, pneumonia might have been called "chronic coughing syndrome." But medical bureaucracy (some call it "biopolitics") moves very slowly, and rarely admits its own errors. So they called it chronic fatigue syndrome back in 1988, and they really don't intend to change it until they have nailed down its causative agent. This is a perfect reason for many in the medical profession to retain their argument that the disease doesn't exist: "We can't find the culprit. There must be nothing wrong."

The arrogance of the implications of that attitude is alarming. Do doctors have *all* the answers? Do they think just because they can't find an answer, there is no question? I can understand the Ford mechanic saying there's nothing wrong with my car because he can't find the source of the engine vibration, but we're talking about *lives*, not cars! What if the FBI denied there had been a bank robbery just because they hadn't found a suspect? "We're sorry, ma'am. We just can't find any robbers so we think the whole thing was in your head. The witnesses, the missing money, that hold-up note, even the pictures on the surveillance camera—they just don't matter. Until we find a suspect, there simply wasn't any crime."

I believe that fatigue is to CFS what homosexuality was to AIDS: It is a place to hide this terrible disease for a while, believing it only affects people who choose a certain life-style. It is that belief that led to the term "yuppie flu" for CFS and "gay cancer" for AIDS. Both terms are sadly flawed. I know CFS patients from every segment of society. And we all know that AIDS is not confined to the homosexual population. It is everybody's problem.

Someday the CDC and NIH will have to admit the same about what they now call chronic fatigue syndrome. It is not a yuppie disease, it is not burn-out, it is not extreme tiredness. It is a serious, life-threatening disease, and it is everybody's problem.

So, what would I call this illness?

I couldn't care less. Just get rid of the "F word."

16

WHY ME?

The medical reporter I mentioned in the last chapter posed another question to me which I remember well: "Do you think of yourself as a victim?"

I really hadn't considered the question before. But the meaning of the word *victim* has gotten so twisted around in recent years that I thought long before I answered.

For example, people who kill other people are often portrayed as victims themselves when they appear before a jury. Often their life's circumstances are presented as "evidence" of why they did what they did. They were victims themselves—that should exclude them from responsibility for their actions.

I told the reporter—with the best smile I could manage—that no, I did not consider myself a victim. A patient, that's all, I told him, but not a victim.

This is not to say that I do not feel terribly victimized by what has happened to me. I hate to use a cliché, but the best years of my life have been taken away from me. That's certainly something to be mad about, and I do get very angry sometimes.

Anger, I've learned, is very constructive. In fact, it's a necessary part of the emotional healing process after a great loss. But considering oneself a victim and dwelling on the self-pity that comes along with that do little to help overcome trauma. The goal of the healing process is acceptance of new circumstances.

Soon after I was cut loose from my career, I vowed I would never become a happy sick person, that I would never accept what had happened to me. Yet if you met me in person, you'd have to conclude that I seem to have reached a sort of standoff with my illness. I might not accept it, but I am living with it, making adjustments for it, getting through it. I am trying to make the most of my life as it is. I guess you could say that CFS and I have reached a temporary ceasefire, a truce.

So how did this come about?

The answer is complex. I present the process here as I experienced it so that patients, or those who care about them, can better understand what must take place in the months and years after a serious illness changes one's life.

Psychologists teach that there are five major steps along the road to acceptance: denial, anger, bargaining, grief, and acceptance. It's important to realize that although the classic model lists these steps in this order, in real life you might skip a step. Or you can come across an emotional trigger which activates or reactivates one of the stages before you're ready for it or after you have already been through it. That happens to me all the time. Just when I think I've licked denial, controlled anger, been through the bargaining, grieved all I can grieve, and am well on the way to acceptance, something comes along and I'm back into it all over again. I doubt that for a chronically ill person, or someone fighting a new disability, the process ever really ends.

I spent more than three years of my illness in denial, thinking that things would eventually work out—they always had before. But denial didn't get me through this continuing ordeal. Denial is a very primitive coping mechanism, and its only real advantage, I suppose, is that it helps us over that initial shock when we learn our world is falling apart.

I had plenty to be angry about—and anger was the next step to deal with. I lost my health, my healthy appearance, much of my intelligence, my perfect memory, my job, my career, my earning power, my responsibilities as the head of my household, my beloved flying, and my friends and staff at the television station who had become a family to me. It seemed as if I'd lost control of my entire life. And to what mighty foe had I lost this all? Probably some tiny virus that could build a sprawling estate on the head of a pin.

I went through many months of bitter anger, sometimes shout-ing at the walls, sometimes crying all alone, sometimes just quietly inventorying all that had been taken away from me. Other times I'd focus on someone who was completely innocent—at my wife or family, usually for something small and insignificant; at friends who didn't call or who didn't seem to care. I regret each of these incidents, and I so wish I could undo them, but like the illness that has racked my body, there seems to be no undoing what is already done. And so I hope and pray that with the people who really mat-ter to me, there is an extra measure of understanding for my behav-ior.

As I mentioned earlier, on the MMPI personality test, CFS patients score in a unique manner. We tip the ends of some scales far beyond what is normal, leading some people to think we are mentally ill. We do not score that way because our illness is in our minds, however, but rather because of a complex series of issues dealing with the mystery, doubt, and frustration surrounding our physical disease. There are people now studying the effects of CFS on the personality, finally putting the cart and the horse in the proper order. For so long, people thought CFS *came from* the mind. In actuality, like any terrible experience, it affects the mind.

Dr. Cheney has come up with an interesting analogy to describe why we all seem to tip certain scales on the MMPI. "Imagine a person who has been placed inside a hole for a year," he once told an interviewer. "They would score quite like a chronic fatigue syndrome patient. They would be angry and in pain, and that would come through in the testing, but that would not mean they are mentally unbalanced."

His analogy is so true. I once told a television interviewer that my existence is like living in a submarine because my illness has taken me so out of touch with real life. I do not experience the things that normal people feel; I do not even record memories. I don't see many sunrises or sunsets, I don't go for walks in the parks, I don't often get to spend relaxing "quality" time with people or do the things I wish I could. That definitely breeds anger that erupts like a volcano at times.

But Dr. Robertson taught me two very important things about

my anger. First, it's okay to be angry. Somehow in my personality development I had become a peacemaker, someone who tried to make everything right in my world. As a result, I had never learned to express anger properly, and all my anger needed to be let out.

Second, he taught me to express my anger in the right direction—at my illness and not at the people and things around me.

Initially I thought of this as psychobabble, some sort of therapy technique. How could I be mad at a list of symptoms or the mysterious cause behind them? I could always smell a rat, and I wasn't about to try some therapy technique or exercise just because it showed up in some trendy new book. Tell me like it is, then I'll deal with it. Don't tell me to imagine a picture of my illness on some pillow and then punch it out! I need more realism than that.

But I began to realize that Robertson's idea wasn't just some sort of technique. (He never suggested punching pillows.) Directing my anger made a lot of sense. It was this disease that had taken everything from me, not the people I knew and cared about. I now work to focus my anger on CFS and not on me or the people around me. That change has made life so much easier. I can enjoy times with my wife, even when I'm feeling bad, even when I'm disappointed about a career on hold or a body that doesn't look anything like it did a few years ago. Misdirected anger is a major obstacle to getting on with a fairly normal life.

The next stage—bargaining—gave me a little trouble. At first I thought it meant that I should be bargaining with God. My own personal faith allows that you can pray—even ask for a miracle—but you don't bargain with God, as in "I'll do this for You, if You do that for me." Even if things work out, humans rarely keep their end of the deal.

Still, it's in our nature to bargain with whom we believe to be our Creator. Looking back, I can see where I did some of this bargaining. When I thought my illness would force me to quit work, I remember praying about my staff and my company. "If only I can keep going for them. . . ."

I think another bargaining point was my writing and communicating ability. I remember seeing the depressing brain map results, wondering how I could ever become a successful writer. I know I asked for divine help then: "Let me do just *this*, and I'll help tell the world the truth about CFS. Maybe I can do some good."

So like other humans going through trials, I made my own bargains with God. I intend to keep my end of the deal, because He kept His. (That statement is more bargaining, you say? Well, I did allow as the process is ongoing!) Even if I were miraculously healed tomorrow, I would still remain loyal to the cause of better understanding for this illness. That's my end of the bargain, and I'm going to keep it.

I didn't even want to go through grieving about what I'd lost—the next step on the list. I was at first repelled by what I considered yet another psychological technique to make me feel a little better. It is hard enough not getting angry all over again when I think about my loss. But slowly I began to take an inventory of my life, of what I'd had and what I'd lost. The anger was quickly replaced by sadness; the grieving had begun.

I looked at videotapes of a handsome weathercaster laughing and smiling, and then looked in the mirror at a very different person. I looked at tapes of my flying everything from Cessnas to the F-16. I pulled out old photos, looked through my logbook to relive old flights, searched through memos and commendations and impressive awards, and read my own articles and sharp quotes in various television and aviation magazines. I thought about the trips Hettie and I used to take to Kennebunkport, to Florida, to the Caribbean. I thought about the great feeling of pushing myself and getting in shape, of attractive women who used to notice me, and of a staff who used to need me. I thought about friends who moved on and moved away, friends that I might never have the ability to see again.

There was, it turned out, plenty to grieve over, and I eventually allowed myself to mourn the loss of each of these things. But as I did, I also counted myself lucky to have had these things in the first place. Not many people my age have had the experiences I've been lucky enough to live. With grief also came a sense of accomplishment and appreciation. Grieving was the most therapeutic of the stages for me to go through, and it did the most to heal my wounded spirit.

The night I spent waiting to be terminated from my job is a good example of constructive grieving. I started out feeling sorry for myself, but ended up feeling good about having had all those things to begin with.

When it came to the final stage—acceptance—I remained a holdout. I had vowed I would never become a happy, well-adjusted sick person—nothing but the old me would ever be acceptable. I would retain the miserable and stubborn attitude that I simply would not accept what had happened to me. I simply would not adapt to what had happened.

Then one day Dr. Robertson substituted the word *integration.*

I hated that word *acceptance.* To me, acceptance meant just taking life as it came. It was a passive notion, and even in this terrible illness, I'm not a passive person. But *integration* is an action word, my kind of word.

And so the challenge had been laid down: Tim Kenny, *integrate* what has happened to you into a new and useful life. It was a plan of action for a man of action.

I recognize that not many CFS patients are as lucky as I am to have had a Dr. Cheney or Dr. Robertson or Janie Warlick or Sheryl Autry or Hettie in their lives. Few have had the hope that Ampligen offered. Many are very much alone. Hundreds, maybe thousands, can't even leave their beds. Some are in wheelchairs, others hardly able to speak.

Writing about my experience, giving television and newspaper interviews, and serving on the board of directors for the world's largest CFS advocacy organization all give me a sense of purpose. Together with the support of the people mentioned above and others, it all provides a reason to keep living, to keep integrating my circumstances into daily living. But many other CFS patients, confined to bed or virtually alone, sense no such purpose and have no such support network.

How can these people complete the process of acceptance, of

coming to terms with their illness? How can they successfully integrate CFS into their lives? How can they find some meaning in their lives, some useful purpose?

To any person anywhere facing personal crisis, I would say realize that you are important, even if you can't contribute financially to the economy, your family, or your own care. Your worth comes from your character, as Dr. Robertson told me so many times, not solely from your job or what you can contribute. It took me years to be able to believe that, so I don't expect anyone to simply accept it on faith. But I'm living proof that it works.

Surround yourself with someone or something that loves you. If you don't have a family or a mate who cares, get a pet. My dogs love me no matter how much money I make or what a jerk I've been. If you can't care for a dog or cat, even a goldfish on your nightstand will make a difference. It'll *need* you, and we all want to feel needed. Find something that thinks you're the greatest, no matter what. For me, thanks to my wife, my family, and my faith, that was already in place, but it's okay if you have to work at it. If you need to, find someone to counsel you through this process. I did, and I probably could not have survived without it.

Allow yourself to feel the anger. Certain therapeutic techniques, although not right for me, may work for you. Scream, punch your pillow, smash a plate, or kick a door (one of my personal favorites). It's okay—even necessary—to be angry.

Don't be afraid to bargain. God might take you up on it, and together you can do good work.

Don't hesitate to grieve, either. Some people call it mourning. If your life is in the grips of CFS, you have much to mourn, much to grieve about. Find pictures of the person you used to be, an old pay stub or W-2 form that recorded your old wages, or anything that reminds you of what you have lost. Allow yourself to experience the sadness. It's natural. It's necessary. And don't be afraid to ask for help anywhere in this process. Chronic fatigue syndrome is a mighty foe that digs deeply into every part of someone's life. Reinforcements come in handy.

If you go through all of these steps, yet refuse to accept the new hand that's been dealt you, consider the concept of integration.

Make a new life from the ashes of the old. You may not be able to give a TV interview or write a book, or even cook dinner on your spouse's birthday, but you are an important person, totally unique in the history of the universe.

The process of learning to face the emotions of serious illness is long and involved. As I did, you may need help during it, but it usually happens quite naturally.

I think one of the most important things you can do is to stop thinking of yourself as a victim and start facing the emotions that will eventually bring about inner peace. It's hard to find peace when you're always asking "Why me?" and feeling sorry for yourself. That will happen from time to time—as it does for me—but don't dwell in self-pity. It's much more productive to confront the issues of denial, anger, bargaining, grief, and integration, and to get on with what's left of your life.

If you or someone you care about is caught in the grip of CFS, embarking on that process may be nearly as important as seeking medical attention. Don't waste valuable time considering the implications of being a victim. Fight this battle straight on, using every fiber of your character. Don't run from it; don't pretend that you're the one who doesn't need to confront this process.

Instead of being a victim, strive to be a victor. Strive to do everything we can to face this terrible disease and come out on top.

17

NEW BEGINNINGS

SCARECROW: *I haven't got a brain, only straw.*
DOROTHY: *How can you talk if you haven't got a brain?*
SCARECROW: *I don't know, but some people without*
brains do an awful lot of talking, don't they?
DOROTHY: *Yes, I guess you're right.*

—From *The Wizard of Oz*

I drove up to the small hospital in Butler, Pennsylvania at about 6:40 P.M. on March 4, 1992. The CFS support group was to meet at seven o'clock. People in wheelchairs and people with canes were already making their way from the parking lot toward the door. Others walked on their own power with an unsteady but determined step.

I felt humbled and afraid because I was their guest speaker, invited to address this group not far from where I had grown up. These people were coming to see me.

I had chosen Butler as the first place to make a CFS speech before an audience for several reasons. First, it was home. I'd be among friends if I should crash and burn. Second, this group was many miles from the halls of information and research that I walked regularly in Charlotte. These people were hungry for information. My regular letters to them were something of an unofficial grapevine about the latest in CFS research. They wanted to hear my story first-person, and I wanted to hear theirs.

And, third, I felt the time had come for me to give back a little of the hope that people like Dr. Cheney, Dr. Robertson, Sheryl Autry, Janie Warlick, Hettie, and others had given to me. In addition, the "blind" had been taken off the Ampligen study, and I knew that I was one of only forty-seven people receiving this drug in its first major clinical trial. I felt that I had a debt to pay, and this was a good place to start paying it.

Dr. Cheney speaks of a resonance when he goes out to talk around the country, and I encountered that very resonance in Pennsylvania that night. Despite the controversy and misunderstanding surrounding this illness, we patients all speak the same language. We've all been through the same experience, the same emotions. As I began to tell my story to this group, I saw heads nod slowly but thankfully in agreement. I saw eyes well up with tears. It is so reassuring to know you are not alone in this fight.

I passed around an empty Ampligen bottle from my infusion earlier in the week. I wanted them all to touch it, to feel it, to believe that it was more than just a concept—that it was real. And I told them how it had brought me back for a season, and how we thought it could bring me back again someday with the proper dosage. Perhaps it could do the same for some of them. Ampligen may not be the answer, it might not be a cure, but it is a sign that someone is trying.

I shared with them a conversation I'd had just two days earlier with Dr. Cheney, especially for them. I conveyed to them his message of hope, that progress was taking place.

I held up an article from a medical journal that Dr. Cheney had sent along with me. The report acknowledged unique hormonal abnormalities in CFS patients, and while it was hardly earth-shattering, it was virgin territory for its authors, the National Institutes of Health.

"It didn't make the headlines," I said, "but this is the first government-written paper that admits CFS is not depression or some other psychiatric illness."

I paused to let the message sink in.

"Do you understand what I'm saying?" I continued. "Finally, the NIH has admitted there *is* an organic basis to this illness.

Though they are years behind the private research, they finally know we are not crazy!"

There were more tears from people who'd waited a long time for some validation of this sort. It was a moving moment. Many— if not most—CFS patients are told more than once that their problems are all in their minds. I've lost count of how many times that was said to me. Vindication is coming slowly, and we grasp for every ounce of it.

I told them of people like Dr. Cheney and others they had read about, and how they were of one mind: to find a cause and a cure, or at least an effective treatment, for CFS.

I had once visited a member of my family at a drug and alcohol rehabilitation center called New Beginnings. There is a sign on the grounds that reads, "At every end, there's a new beginning." While he was at New Beginnings, I had also sent my relative a quote from Louis L'Amour's *Lonely on the Mountain:* "There will come a time when you believe everything is finished. That will be the beginning." I shared those quotes with the group in Butler that evening, as I experienced something of a new beginning myself.

There in that small Pennsylvania hospital where I'd had my lip sewn up years earlier following a gym class collision and where I'd had several other parts of my body stitched up over the years, another patch job took place that night. I found my own new beginning, after many months of searching. I found a place to start to make some sense out of my own ashes.

I vowed that night that I'd begin by trying to reach other patients with the message of hope that was so apparent back in Charlotte, but seemed so far away here in a small Pennsylvania hospital.

I came home from there determined to write this book, determined to speak to any group that will listen to me.

I closed the meeting in Butler by reading the essay that appears below. I had written it a short time before the meeting, one of the dozens of essays I wrote during the period in which I was confronting my illness and the realities it had brought me. That period was one of daily emotional upheaval and self-discovery. Little did I realize that the stories I was writing—many seemingly about things other than my illness—were actually metaphors for the process that was taking place within me. The steps that I had been told about—denial, anger, bargaining, grief, and integration—slowly revealed themselves to me in my own writing—in stories about my dogs, my flying, my acquaintances, and my experiences. They were in a very real sense stories that illustrated my own emotional healing process, no matter what their subject.

CLIMBING FOR THE SUNSHINE

A gray rainy sky hung over the entire Southeast as I prepared for one of my earliest flying trips, the first leg of which would be aboard a small, noisy commuter airliner. It would be a long time before I became a pilot myself, so I quickly prejudged the propeller-driven aircraft and its crew as second-class citizens in the world of aviation. Now I know better, for those planes are worth millions of dollars—even if they do have propellers on their wings—and the flight crew must meet rigid standards of proficiency, the same as their jet-flying counterparts.

But I knew none of this then, and I suppose I imagined that this part of aviation—to which I had not been exposed in the past—was something of a secret from the authorities.

Through the steadily falling rain, we taxied out from the single-gate terminal to the active runway.

After a few minutes of preflight checks, the pilots advanced the two throttles and we were soon bucking our way down the runway. Even though the plane was old and loud and seemingly not worthy of my trust, I remember the feeling of acceleration pressing me ever so slightly back into my seat. Then in a moment, we were airborne, and the bumping and jarring of the runway were beneath us.

For such a rainy day, I was surprised to find that the sky itself held few bumps. We climbed smoothly into the rain clouds as I resigned myself to the fact that the view out my window—rain, a wing, and a propeller—would be all the view I'd enjoy on this trip.

But suddenly, about ten minutes later, something totally unexpected happened.

With no warning whatsoever, that despised little airplane seemed to pop from the tops of the clouds and we were immediately basked in the most brilliant sunshine I could have imagined. I knew next to nothing about weather back then, so I guess I assumed that the dreariness of that Sunday afternoon reached infinitely toward the heavens and that there was no escaping its grip no matter how high we climbed.

But how wrong I was! How I thrilled at being in such shimmering sun when the dreary world below was being drenched. Aboard a plane I didn't trust or really believe in, we had climbed above the weather for this part of our flight, and it was a victorious half-hour that I'll always remember.

Many years later, after I had become a pilot, I worked harder still and earned an instrument rating, the license that allows pilots to fly through clouds and other weather that restricts visibility. I myself now had the power to climb above some overcast skies and some dreary Sundays, though my experience and pocketbook didn't usually allow me access to the kinds of aircraft needed to fly high enough. Once or twice, though, I was blessed with being at the controls when it happened. I know that if you'd been flying beside me, you'd have seen a little boy's smile cross the pilot's face at the moment we spurted forth into the sunshine.

Most of the time I experienced that wonderful event, it was aboard a jet airliner where I was just a passenger. But even then I marvelled at the realization that sunshine and clear skies are always above somewhere, no matter how lousy the weather is on the ground.

Twice I was invited to fly in the supersonic F-16 Falcon, which climbs at a rate greater than thirty thousand feet per minute. Though the actual top altitude the F-16 can attain is classified by the Air Force, I doubt there is a rainy day anywhere that it can't outclimb in less than two minutes. Ah, if life were only so easy!

Today as I write, it's another dreary Sunday afternoon. The weather forecast says it will remain that way all day, with clearing later in the week. And today as I write, there are aspects of my own life that seem every bit as dreary as this day. And in my life there is no extended forecast promising sunshine in a few days, if only I can hang on.

But I must remember that noisy commuter airplane, the times I myself flew through nasty weather, and the exhilarating feeling of going vertical in an F-16 faster than a bullet and popping out into the crystal blue sky, surrounded by the beauty of sunshine that was hidden to me back on the ground. And I must remember that airplanes climb much more slowly than they cruise. At times, especially in a headwind, one's progress seems almost nonexistent.

I must remember to keep trying to climb above this dreariness—above the rain and the gray. I must keep looking upward for the lighter clouds, a sure sign that the sunshine is only a few hundred feet higher.

There are times when I don't want to trust this vessel that I'm traveling in. Like the noisy and ragged commuter plane of a decade ago, there are reasons why that would be the natural thing to do. But the call of the clear blue sky, the promise of sunshine again, is enough—for this moment at least—to keep me going.

And so I plod onward through the rain and the gray, at speeds so slow they are almost immeasurable, barely clinging to flight and sustained only by the hope that—above all of this—there is a sunny day somewhere, just waiting for me to find it.

18

THE ARCHITECTURE
OF SURVIVAL

A Story About Denial

It was from the chief engineer of WPDE that I first learned about the architecture of survival. It's not a notion I would have thought of, but technology and humanity alike owe it much.

We were at our giant broadcasting tower, a steel structure weighing millions of pounds and stretching two thousand feet into the air. This tower is so big that there's an elevator that runs right through the center of it. The concrete that forms its base and support anchors could have built a parking lot or a medium-size building. There are literally miles of guy wires holding each section carefully in place. To stand anywhere near this tower makes me marvel at the engineering accomplishment that allows it to exist at all and to not be crushed beneath its own weight. Contrary to what I had thought, anything as massive as this tower, many times higher than the Statue of Liberty and easily dwarfing the Empire State Building, anything this big must be almost alive to survive.

All the weight of that tremendous structure rests on a single common point. The base of the tower forms a V with an immeasurably strong ball at its very bottom, fitting into a saucer-like receptacle.

It's not what I would have expected to find at the bottom of the tower, so I asked the engineer about it.

"That's so it can move," he told me.

"*Move?*" I queried, incredulous. "Why do you want it to move?"

"Otherwise it'd blow over or break," he answered. "It's gotta be strong enough to stand up, but it's gotta have enough give to twist and sway. Otherwise," he said, climbing easily into the elevator car, "it could just snap right off."

And with that he was gone up the tower, a two-thousand-foot trip that takes twenty minutes each way.

I had thought that the massive structure would be rigid at the bottom to prevent any twisting and moving. I guess that's why I don't design or build towers.

Then, I thought about the 1989 San Francisco earthquake. The Nimitz Freeway viaduct, the solid concrete-and-steel structure built hard and firm the way I would build it, was the structure that collapsed. The marvelous Golden Gate Bridge, hanging over the bay by those steel ropes, literally swinging and swaying every second, held strong throughout the earthquake.

Since I grew up near Pittsburgh, where there are three rivers, I got to drive on plenty of bridges. I can attest to the fact that those big suspension bridges sway quite a bit, especially if you're stuck in traffic on one. But someone told me that the sway was actually engineered into the bridge, and it was when they stopped swaying that I should worry.

This nonrigid technology is used in other places. The city of Tokyo, one of the most populous places per square mile on earth, sits squarely on a huge earthquake fault. In the early 1900s, a massive earthquake leveled the city. Now, all of the buildings have to be earthquake-proof.

So how do you make a building earthquake-proof? By giving it the ability to sway, to move, to be alive when the earth beneath it begins to slide and shake.

I'm still not completely comfortable with this concept, though I have come to accept it as fact. And so it was recently, as I drove through the rolling hills a hundred or so miles from my home, that I spotted a broadcasting tower and started thinking again about this whole process of swaying. I had no idea I would witness it in the world's most incredible engineering achievement of all—humanity—in only a few hours.

We were at a friend's home, watching a movie, when a call came in about an acquaintance of our friend who had been in a terrible car accident and who, several hours later, had still not regained consciousness. Soon, we were at the hospital to find out the latest information and lend our support.

There were more than a dozen friends and co-workers gathered in the emergency room hallway. A tired and discouraged doctor appeared to bring everyone up to date.

"I'm afraid I don't have any good news," he began, looking at the feet of the people gathered hopefully around him. "Her brain is terribly swollen," he explained, adding that it was so damaged this young schoolteacher wasn't even able to breathe for herself. When a person's brain cannot even make the rest of the body tend to its need for blood and oxygen, the prognosis is indeed bad.

"There's really nothing I can do," he concluded. "Her parents should be in town by morning. I hope we can keep her alive until then."

Although I had never met this woman, I wanted to chase the doctor's words back into his throat. "No, you can't be saying it's over, that she's dying," I wanted to say. "That just can't be so!"

But it was so, and her friends that had gathered in that place to wait and hope and pray began to break into smaller groups and comfort each other as best they could.

I wondered what I'd do if I had known her, if the doctor had been speaking to me about someone I knew and loved. I think I know the answer, though I hope I never find out. I think I would have somehow, some way, snapped. I would have tried to remain firm and strong and rigid, and would have broken as surely as a rigid structure would when confronted by the unimaginable forces of nature. I would have crumbled and become useless, because I could not accept the terrible blow that fate had just dealt.

In my own life I am facing a crisis today, though thankfully it is not a crisis of life and death. It is a crisis of great loss, though, and I know that in order to get on with what remains of my life, I must not stay in this terrible stage of denial; I must not remain rigid. I need to bend and sway under the terrible weight of what is happening to me, and I must go on from here. I can learn a great deal from that group of strangers I saw in the hospital corridor the night the young schoolteacher died.

As I write this, nearly twenty-four hours have passed since the doctor's announcement in that hallway. The young woman with so many strong friends died about six hours after the doctor spoke those words. Then the miracles began.

People began to think about her family and her friends at home in another state. They began to care for her dog, and make arrangements for her apartment and her belongings. They picked out the clothing for her to be buried in, and they tended to dozens of other details. And they stayed together. They were stunned and shocked and saddened beyond what it would seem the human spirit should have to endure, but they withstood the shock, steadied each other, and went on with what had to be done.

I know there are dozens, perhaps even hundreds, of people who have been touched by this tragedy. And I marvel at them all, with much more admiration than I have for a bridge or a building or a TV tower, but an admiration born of what such structures have taught me. For in their loss and in their grief, they have allowed themselves to comfort and be comforted, to cry and to hurt, and to go on with what must be done.

They are able to do it because that tiny group of tearful people outside the emergency room sagged at the knees and swayed, ever so slightly and for only a passing moment, the way all of us must learn to do if we are to survive life's most crushing blows.

19

THE WISDOM TO KNOW THE DIFFERENCE
A Story About Anger

Back when I was the news director for a network affiliate television station, I was a pretty busy person. But I wasn't too busy to notice the look on Robert's face the last day he worked for us.

Robert was a master control switcher, the person who played all the tapes and commercials and made sure the shows got on the air. He'd been at the station since its first year of operation. He was leaving the station now to go to truck-driving school, after years of punching buttons in the dimly lit master control room. No one could blame him. He'd put in many years at the boring master control console—that would be enough to make anyone long for the open road.

After his final shift on the final day with us, I spotted Robert sort of aimlessly roaming the halls in a part of the television station where master control switchers are rarely seen. I knew what he was doing.

"Hard to believe it will go on without you, isn't it?" I asked, as Robert leaned into the room where the graphic artist worked.

"Huh?" he responded, somewhat startled that he'd been noticed.

"You've been here so long and been so much a part of everything that you kind of wish things would stop for a minute while you leave, right?"

"I guess that's what I'm feeling," Robert admitted.

"Or at least maybe you wish things would at least slow down," I went on.

Robert nodded.

We walked to my office and we both sat down.

"It can't happen that way," I said, stating the obvious. "Remember when Radar O'Reilly left M*A*S*H?" I asked. Of course Robert did, because he'd played every episode of the show as reruns on our station. "There were incoming wounded, and all the staff was so busy trying to save lives that when the time came for Radar to get on the chopper, all they could do was look up from their work and nod a quick goodbye. There weren't hugs and parties or anything. Life went on because it had to, and Radar would have wanted it that way, even though a part of him wanted it to all stop when he left."

Robert was quiet now, recalling the episode I mentioned. Robert remembered every show he'd ever played on the air. After about a minute, he spoke. "I guess I know what you mean," he said slowly. "I know that the station has to go on, and I know it'll go on without me. But I do kind of wish that my leaving would make a difference."

"Your being here is what made the difference," I told him. "Leaving is a natural part of life. You'll be missed, but everyone is so busy with their jobs right now, that you're not going to get much of a send-off. Don't feel bad about that," I continued. "You did your job well, and you helped train your replacement. That, as much as anything, is a tribute to the years you put in here."

A new look crossed Robert's face, and we shook hands as he turned to leave, both of us feeling a little better about his departure.

That was a few years ago, when I had begun to fight an illness that I then knew nothing about. I certainly didn't know that my illness would cause me to leave my job for a reason less joyful than Robert's. There was no open road calling me—only hours of loneliness and pain and the terrible feeling of being left behind by a world that had better things to do.

In the time since I have gotten off the world, it has continued, much to my dismay, to turn exactly as it did before. The first day of winter came right on schedule, Christmas and New Year's Day went on as planned, and my television station kept going just as the surgeons of the 4077th kept operating as Radar looked his goodbyes through the operating room window.

But that doesn't mean I have to be happy about it, and it doesn't mean I can't feel what Robert felt on his last day a thousand times over.

One of the hardest parts for me has been seeing the people that I hired or trained or guided in some way leave for bigger and better things. Sure, that's what I always wanted for them, but back then I thought the world held bigger and better things for me, too. Now I am not at all sure about that.

Tommy—my best friend and my weathercaster—is now in Columbus, Ohio, where he is becoming more popular every day. He's on a fast-moving train toward the top of his profession.

Amanda, someone hard for me to get close to but someone I picked right out of college as a future star, is now working far away in Portland, Maine, one of the most beautiful northeastern cities I know, and a great place for the second step in her career.

Bill, my former boss from the days of Hurricane Hugo, left to run a big station in Pennsylvania, where he has enough to do without thinking about me. I always thought when Bill moved on, he'd take me with him.

And Sue, someone to whom I once was very close and could blurt out whatever came to mind, left for her hometown of Kansas City to be an anchor. It's quite a step, and something both she and I could be very proud of. Only I had real trouble being happy or proud.

Sue called and invited me to dinner the next-to-last night she was in town. We hadn't spoken for some weeks, and I had a lot to tell her. I wanted to explain to her that I was afraid of being alone, without even one of my old friends around, and I wasn't happy that the last of them was about to leave. I wanted to explain that while she was celebrating and being congratulated, I was struggling with Social Security and disability insurance claims and wondering how I'd pay the mortgage. More than all of that, though, I wanted to say that I needed people to support me, to encourage me, and to help prop up my sagging spirits, while she needed high-fives and going-away cards. Although I wanted to see her one last time, it didn't sound like the recipe for a great time.

Still, I was hoping she could reach through all of what I had to say and the dinner invitation would stand. Only I didn't get to say all of those things.

"Damn you for leaving me!" I heard myself say before the phone line went dead.

She hung up on me, and I suppose I don't blame her. It was hardly the upbeat send-off she'd expected, and it certainly wasn't the encouragement-seeking explanation I thought I would offer. It was the voice of fear, of loneliness, of frustration, and of selfishness.

I know it was the voice of selfishness because I should be angry at this illness, not at people like Sue who continue to live their lives. I should be angry at a virus that has randomly chosen to attack me and end my career, not at friends who are quite naturally continuing their careers. I shouldn't be angry at Tommy for moving to Columbus, at Amanda for moving to a place where you can get twin lobster for about ten dollars, at Bill for moving back to his hometown, or at Sue for moving back to hers. They've all moved on for more money, more prestige, and more responsibility and respect than they had before. I should be proud that our lives were fortunate enough to intersect for a short while, and that we enriched each other, through the good times and the bad.

I should be feeling that way, and I'm working on it, against the deadline of possibly turning all my friends away from me when I need them most. I feel like Radar peering through the operating room window, or Robert roaming the halls.

How can the world continue so easily without me? It doesn't seem fair. But I guess I need to learn to accept some of the terms that have been dealt me. If I don't, I'll do nothing but build a wall between me and the people I care about, and it'll be a wall much thicker than the miles that now separate us.

As the seeds I have sown are cast into the wind, as the people whom I have helped climb their career ladders, I am being left behind. And I'm angry about it and sad about it. I'm tired of everyone else saying goodbye to me, and I'm tired of watching the world go on without me. But I have enough sense to know it's not going to stop for my problems, and it's not even going to slow down to reach out to me. I know in my heart I need to stop being angry at people.

Getting to where I am today was not my choice. How I'll deal with the anger, hurt, and loneliness I'm feeling is my choice. As I peer through the tiny window I have on life, and friends and former co-workers have only the time to look up and nod, I must remember that it's this illness—not their success—that has hurt me so much. I can speak with the voice of fear and loneliness and frustration, and even at times with a small amount of selfishness, but never to the extent that it drives away the very people I need most of all.

I can sit at the keyboard and write about this valuable lesson along my life's journey, but I have yet to learn the lesson completely.

God grant me the wisdom to know the difference.

20

WAKE UP, BOY, YOU CAN SLEEP WHEN YOU'RE DEAD!

A Story About Bargaining

My friend Tom Sorrells sat across the living room from me looking as if he'd been through World War III. Dark circles hugged his sagging eyes, and his skin had a grayish-yellow color. It was 7:30 on a Sunday night, and in just a few minutes I'd be taking Tom to the airport and the flight that would take him home.

Tom had left WPDE about six months before flying in this weekend for a friend's wedding. Tom was more than just a weathercaster; he was really a major personality, the kind of guy who got all the girls, but whom mothers actually wanted their daughters to marry. He had remained a bachelor through his rise to local TV stardom. A big station in Columbus, Ohio had offered big money to lure my best friend away, and this was only his second weekend visit back to his old stomping grounds.

I had picked him up at the airport Friday night and loaned him my car for the weekend. I didn't have any plans, and I wasn't feeling well enough to try keeping up with Tom. By the time he brought my car back Sunday night, he looked like a man definitely in need of rest, and I told him so.

"Aw, I know," he said with the punchiness that comes from three days without sleep, "but I can sleep when I'm dead."

"Where'd that expression come from?" I asked. "Where did you ever hear that about 'you can sleep when you're dead?'"

"When I was a kid," Tom began, his bloodshot eyes rolling back to extract memory. "My dad used to bang on my door early Saturday mornings to get me moving. He usually had work around the house he wanted me to do, and he'd holler, 'Wake up, boy, you can sleep when you're dead!'"

His dad had a point.

Another friend of mine, a guy named Charlie, told me stories about how he used to drive from Charlotte to the Outer Banks of North Carolina for a weekend of fishing when he was a few years younger.

"We'd fish the whole weekend," Charlie mused.

"Well, not the whole weekend," I tried to correct him. "Where'd you sleep? Right on the beach?"

"Sleep?" Charlie asked. "Hell, man, I didn't drive all that way to sleep. I drove there to fish, and that's what I did!"

This was something of a new concept to me.

I spent a short time of my early working life selling furniture, and always enjoyed selling mattresses. "You spend a third of your life sleeping," I'd remind customers as they looked at the price ticket. A good mattress and box spring set can run as high as seven or eight hundred dollars, and I would need a line like that to help the customer get over sticker shock. Guys like Tommy and Charlie, though, kind of blew that theory for me. Here were a couple of guys who knew a chance for fun and adventure when they saw it, and wouldn't let something as simple as sleep get in their way.

I've been rethinking this theory of sleep lately, and I believe I'm getting closer to Tommy and Charlie's way of looking at things. I used to go a day or two without sleep when work demanded it, such as when I worked at the television station, but I never passed on sleep simply to enjoy a little more out of life. I'd only done it when I had no other choice.

I'm not in television anymore. I feel like I'm not in anything. I'm sick, and they say until they get this all figured out, I can't work anymore. I have to agree with them, but that doesn't mean I'm taking the news—if you'll pardon the pun—lying down.

While trying to figure out what's going on, the doctors ran a sophisticated brain scan on me. The scan said I was *asleep*; only I wasn't. I was awake; I was reading, talking, thinking, even doing some simple calculations. But the machine said the predominant wave in my brain right now, especially when I close my eyes, is the sleep wave, and everything else in my brain is running on only three cylinders. The doctors really can't understand how I get around, let alone manage to think and laugh and occasionally remember to write them a check.

Well, that's for them to figure out.

I've asked for some divine help fighting that sleep wave and trying to take this time getting the best look at life I've ever gotten, since there's not much else to do. I'd be lying if I said it was easy, because it's not. My brain and my body aren't as cooperative as I'd like. This is a real-life example of the biblical saying, "The spirit is willing but the flesh is weak."

But I figure it this way: As long as I keep my eyes open as much as possible, as long as I'm always looking around, I'll keep on seeing things and remembering things. And since just about all I can manage to do is make my way to the computer once or twice a week to type these observations, I'll really be keeping my eyes open, and maybe I'll see or remember a few things that the rest of the world (Tommy and Charlie excluded) are too busy to see.

I guess in the big scheme of things, one more guy walking the earth trying to extract the little bits of life that often go overlooked isn't that big a deal. But for me, it's all I've got. As long as the good Lord above lets me, I'm going to keep looking, keep noticing, and keep writing about things.

After all, Tommy's dad said it best: I can sleep when I'm dead.

21
HIGHEST FLIGHT
A Story About Grieving

I can't believe this is happening, but that is totally understandable. One is rarely prepared to live out his ultimate fantasy, I am certain.

I'm harnessed inside the stretched cockpit of a General Dynamics F-16 fighter. Not just any F-16, mind you, but an F-16 of the elite United States Air Force Aerial Demonstration Squadron—the famous Thunderbirds.

To fly with the Thunderbirds, to ride in an F-16, is a privilege not normally reserved for mere mortals. Somehow, this is my second invitation, and my "experience" in the F-16, plus my own flying credentials, earn me the promise that I can do most of the driving this time around. The regular pilot, a major, will handle the takeoff.

Twenty seconds into the flight, I begin to think that this might not be such a good idea after all. Suddenly, we're absolutely vertical, going straight up, traveling faster than a bullet. My head is spinning. My back and shoulders are plastered against the seat, yet I feel as if I'm about to fall from the sky. My stomach is somewhere several thousand feet below me. You can't live too long without a stomach, I think.

"How we doin'?" the pilot asks as we pierce the cloud layer and spurt into the brilliant sunlight that no one on the ground would see this day.

How we doin'? These jet jockeys *do* have ice water in their veins.

A few seconds later (it doesn't take long to go far at these speeds), we're six miles out over the Atlantic Ocean. Thankfully, we are in level flight at last. Upside-down.

I've never quite trusted airplanes because of a very basic concern deep inside me: If something goes terribly wrong, it's thousands of feet to the ground.

In a moment, my mistrust fades, and I open my eyes to a world that takes my breath away. The ocean is *above* me, and I stare at its bluish beauty dotted by white wisps of wavecaps. I decide that there is no room for fear on this flight; I will completely trust the F-16, even upside-down.

Major Ice Water offers to show me some maneuvers before I take over the stick. We do a perfect loop, using eight thousand feet of altitude, flawlessly connecting our circle of air-show smoke at the bottom. We roll the jet over and over, four times in six seconds. We fly the jet on its side, daring the laws of physics to pluck us from the sky.

Now I am flying, and the maneuvers come easily in this incredible aircraft. Computers compensate for my lack of skill, so my own loops and rolls are impressive, too.

The minutes pass too quickly, and the pilot asks if there is anything else I'd like to do before he takes over for one final stunning maneuver.

Yes, I tell him, there is something I'd like to do. Something generations of men and women have dreamed of, and something that is now a tantalizing possibility.

I want to play in the clouds.

He says okay, and I hear the great jet's engine respond as if to my very thoughts.

I aim for a saddle in a giant billowing cumulus cloud and I am suddenly there. With a tug of my wrist I snap the jet sharply around the anvil-shaped top of the cloud and point the speeding craft at a pristine valley between two more plumes.

In this valley, the air is brilliantly clear, the sunlight radiates with a heavenly brightness, and the world as I knew it seems a million miles distant. At six hundred miles an hour, darting among the clouds is as easy as playing hopscotch.

My pilot and I had struck a deal before we took off, and the time has come to do it. We'll execute a maneuver that'll put us through nine times the force of gravity; as fighter pilots say, "We'll pull nine Gs." My top gun has saved this rarely offered chance until last.

The F-16 is the only jet in the world that can sustain such a load. A pilot must have a tremendous amount of training simply to remain conscious during this experience.

Yes, I feel up to it! What stomach? When will I ever get this chance again? And should I die at this moment, I'll die happy. We agree to go for the nine Gs.

"Airspeed up. We're going to the left," Major Ice Water says calmly. "And heeere we go!"

The F-16 banks sharply as a giant force tugs at my insides, threatening to rip my organs from their assigned positions. My cheeks are dragged downward, leaving a gap below my sagging eyeballs. I see life as I did in the 1960s, in black and white, before we got a color TV set.

We're flying in a tunnel now, and someone must have put a heavy barrel of water on my head. Some of the water is leaking into my eyes; the rest is forcing my head into my lap. My face is vibrating back and forth like a poor comedian's Richard Nixon impression. My spine is being compressed like a collapsible radio antenna.

Other than that, I'm fine.

As we come out of the maneuver, the pilot tells me I have just done something that virtually no nonmilitary aviator ever will. Nine Gs would rip civilian airplanes to pieces.

Fifteen minutes later, we are on the ground.

As we taxi up to the crowd of mechanics, photographers, and others, I'm already discussing the flight as if it were just a walk around the block. Alongside the jet, Major Ice Water presents me with the coveted nine-G pin, which remains one of my most prized possessions.

More than two years have passed since I handled the controls of the F-16 that morning. My flight log book shows only two uneventful flights since then. My health was slipping away well before the Thunderbirds' invitation came. Now, unhappily, I can fly no longer.

I read the notation in my log book which records this incredible experience. For a moment I'm saddened by the empty lines on the remainder of the page, the empty pages that follow. These are flights that never happened, and for all I know may never happen.

But I hold the nine-G pin in my fingers and the sadness disappears. I think of great men like Moses, Da Vinci, the Wright brothers. These were people who looked to the skies, but could only dream of the adventures the heavens contained.

I seek out the writing of John Gillespie Magee, a young American who enlisted in the Royal Canadian Air Force in late 1940, well before the United States entered World War II. Magee was eager to defend Great Britain—his mother's homeland—and he turned down a Yale scholarship to train as a fighter pilot. He died when his plane went down just four days after Pearl Harbor.

On the back of a letter to his parents, Magee had composed the poem "High Flight":

Oh! I have slipped the surly bonds of Earth
And danced the skies on laughter-silvered wings;
Sunward I've climbed, and joined the tumbling mirth
of sun-split clouds,—and done a hundred things
You have not dreamed of—wheeled and soared and swung
High in the sunlit silence. Hov'ring there,
I've chased the shouting wind along, and flung
My eager craft through footless halls of air . . .

Up, up the long, delirious, burning blue
I've topped the windswept heights with easy grace
Where never lark, or ever eagle flew—
And, while with silent lifting mind I've trod
The high untrespassed sanctity of space,
Put out my hand, and touched the face of God.

The words of this brave young man—so eager to defend freedom that he volunteered and gave his life before it was even considered patriotic to do so—forever stir in my heart my own wonderful flying memories.

Once again I feel the awe and spectacle of flight as few will ever feel it, recalling what we did that day in the F-16. I don't need an airplane to make the experience complete—I simply close my eyes. I think about the loops, the rolls, the nine incredible Gs.

I replay the part where—with just the slightest movement of my right wrist—I'm again darting among the clouds in perhaps the world's greatest airplane. What a dream! It's glorious now, as it was then, and on this flight of my imagination, I'll make up for the part I forgot to do before.

Yes, I have done things most people can only dream about, but I do have some unfinished business. There is something John Magee did that I now want to do before I finally agree to abide by gravity's laws, perhaps forever.

In my mind, I point the F-16 at the top of a cloud and spear it perfectly, emerging again into the heavenly sunlight. The air is clear, the sky is brilliant blue, and for a fleeting moment, gravity is not an issue.

As I snap the roaring F-16 around the flowering crown of a towering cumulus cloud, I am at one with the sky and I do not resist the urge to put out my hand.

And this time, I touch the face of God.

From the depths of my grief, miles from the nearest airport, I have just experienced the greatest flight of my life.

The surly bonds of sadness could not hold me.

22

APPLE TREES, TIME TRAVEL, AND THE USS *ENTERPRISE*
A Story About Integration

In just a few hours, I will be heading for the airport and my own home hundreds of miles away, but I have awakened this morning in my parents' home in the very bedroom I occupied two decades earlier. This brief visit has been a step back in time for me, as I have walked the halls of my old school, seen my old teachers with their graying hair, and driven on the back roads that hold so many of my secret memories.

I have saved the most important experience until last, until this morning. It is really not such a big deal. I'm just going to take a walk.

A very intelligent person has told me that in order to deal with my current situation, in order to recognize that I have some value as a person even though I am not working, I must go back to the days when I was younger and find the spot where I got on the fast-moving treadmill that has been my life for so long.

Maybe this walk around the five acres that make up my parents' property will lead me back to that person I was. Maybe it will take me back to being a kid, or just lead me to the part of being a kid that recognizes it's okay just to do nothing once in a while. Doing nothing is my primary occupation these days, and it doesn't seem okay to me.

I leave the house and head out across the back yard, the gravel driveway, and into the area where huge oak trees have deposited a blanket of golden leaves. First I pause at the spot where my beagle used to live. I paid fifteen dollars for her and she brought me a million dollars' worth of happiness. I wish now—now that she is long gone—that I had spent more time with her. I smile, though, at the memories of what we did together, and while it is warming to recall her and our time together, I know this is not what I have set out to find.

I walk to the left to the space where the sheep barn used to stand, and I remember Patches, the small lamb that I raised so that she could one day raise her own lambs. I fed her from a baby bottle until she was old enough to eat the mash that came in the dusty burlap sacks. This, too, is a fond memory, but it is not what I am searching for.

I continue walking. Will there be something I see, something I feel, something I touch or hear that will take me back twenty years?

I walk quickly past the garden. There are no good memories here, and there is no garden here any longer.

I am heading toward the chicken house when I pause at a small bluff and remember Spunky. I don't suppose many people have pet chickens, but Spunky was all I had sometimes, and we would sit together on that bluff and wait for the sun to set and the day to end. She was not entirely healthy, and I suppose that's why she became a pet and not a meal. We would sit on the bluff and she would lay her head across my lap when I was convinced no other living creature in the world would want to be close to me. Now that I am not entirely healthy, I appreciate her caring gesture all the more. It is pleasant to recall Spunky, and I can see her plainly in my mind's eye. Again, I am warmed by the memory and thankful for it, but I am still not sure that this is what I have been looking for.

From this bluff I leave the thoughts of my pet chicken and head toward the chicken house. It was built of ancient used lumber twenty years earlier, so it looks a century old now as I walk up the concrete steps. The warped door no longer wants to open, but I force it and make my way inside. Now the coop merely houses junk, but over the years hundreds of chickens relied on me for their daily staples in this building. On the wall to the right I remember where the boxes were built for the young pullets to lay their first eggs, and I remember the mysterious thrill of retrieving the eggs each day. My memories are foggy, but surely there had to be a way for the chickens to get outside. I move some of the clutter, and there is the hole in the wall that I myself had cut so that the chickens could spend their days outside, and return at night to roost. The hole is irregular and misshapen, attesting to my skills as a carpenter, then and now.

I suddenly remember the rafters and my hiding place. Wasn't there a ladder? I turn around and see it, boards nailed to the northern wall, though the bottom rungs are gone. I am disappointed, sure my weakened arms cannot pull me up without those first steps. Or can they? When will I ever get this chance again? With the midmorning sun filtering through wire-covered windows, I grasp for the high rungs and pull myself upward. It is a struggle, and if this ancient wood gives way, I am in big trouble. In a moment, though, I am sitting on the rafters, looking down into the chicken house like so many years ago. I look around at the rusted chicken feeders and water troughs stored up here. Though the memory of my hiding place was worth the effort to get up here, even this place does not provide whatever it is I am seeking today. I still have not found the youngster who lived in this body and who could be happy without even thinking about a career or a paycheck.

I swing from the rafters and my feet land back on the floor, sending up a shower of two-decade-old dust. I leave the henhouse and continue my time travel.

I am at the pond now; only this year it is dry. I remember that one day I buried a pet here, though my clouded mind cannot remember which one. I also remember how I sunk the aircraft carrier USS *Enterprise* in this pond. I spent days, maybe weeks, building the *Enterprise* from a Tyco model kit, and I labored over painting each of the tiny jets on her flight deck. For some reason (probably my brother's urging), she had to go down in flames. With the help of some M-80s and a cup of gasoline, the *Enterprise* slipped beneath the water of the pond two decades earlier, black smoke marking the spot of her grave. I don't know the life span of Tyco model plastic, but I imagine it to be much longer than twenty years, and I guess that if I went poking around in the reeds that now grow where the pond once was, I will find the blackened hull. I don't bother, though, because, while I am still not sure of what I am looking for, I am certain it is not the *Enterprise*.

I begin to head back toward the house, several hundred yards distant now, and detour slightly to a field where I once lifted eighty-pound bales of fresh hay and learned the real meaning of hard work. I can almost smell the freshly cut clover of two decades ago.

My father has gone for a walk this morning, too, and we meet in his apple orchard. Apples are his favorite subject, and though I wanted to be alone on this trip back through time, I strike up an apple conversation with him.

"What are those things that look like cowbells hanging from some of the branches?" I ask him.

"Weights," he says, "to keep the trees from growing upward."

I am confused. "I thought you wanted the trees to grow big," I tell him.

"No, no, no!" he goes on, as if I should somehow know this already. "If the branch goes up, the enzymes say grow, but if the branch is held down, the enzymes say make more fruit." He is then on to another apple topic, but I am not ready to leave this one.

"So you actually hold the branches down?" I ask. My dad has strange ideas about many things, and I press him to see if this is just another such notion. It is not, he assures me, his idea, but has been practiced for centuries. Some orchards employ wires to hold the branches down, others have stakes in the ground to which the branches are tied. The latest idea from scientists at a major university is the cowbell-shaped weights.

"Okay," I say. "The tree wants to grow up big and tall, but if it does, it won't make much fruit, right? But if you hold it down—limiting its growth—it won't concentrate on growing, but it will concentrate on making more fruit? Is that how it works?"

"You got it," my dad says, and is off on some story about how a hired helper killed some trees with too much pesticide. I'm not listening, though, because I'm thinking about the branches that want to reach for the sky, but can't, only to produce even more fruit in their frustration. Suddenly, thinking of my own situation, how I want to reach for the sky but cannot, I realize that I have something in common with those apple trees. And I think that maybe now—now that I cannot grow big and tall and be a successful broadcaster—maybe now I can somehow take this time to bear some kind of fruit, something that will be of real value to someone. It is an abstract notion, to be sure, but when one is seeking a reason to continue living, to face another empty day, one will look anywhere, and nature is not such a bad place to start. I have not been struck by lightning nor had some instant conversion experience, but I am sure I will not forget the story about the apple trees.

Three hours later I am on a jet heading south, watching West Virginia slip by beneath me. The mountains are so beautiful in this crisp fall afternoon that I have for a while forgotten about my walk through time, and I've have just been enjoying the scenery. Then I see an orchard on the side of a mountain beneath me and I am reminded of my journey earlier in the day.

I still do not know what I was looking for on that walk, and so I do not believe I actually found it. But somehow, I think, considering the lesson of the apple trees, I have not come away empty-handed.

23

THE SPARK THAT KEEPS
ME GOING

I shivered against the biting wind, my numbing fingers trying to attach a two-foot microwave antenna to its portable receiver. I was atop the Palace Hotel, Myrtle Beach's tallest building, on the final night of winter 1990, and Mother Nature wasn't about to let the season end peacefully.

This was the eve of Hurricane Hugo's six-month anniversary, and that was why I was working after sunset in the bitter blowing cold. I had been diagnosed with CFS just three weeks earlier and I was still deep in denial, far from taking my doctor's advice to slow down, still trying to prove I could do it all.

Our television station was going to do a special program about the recovery from Hugo the following night, and I was trying to establish a portable microwave station that would allow us to transmit from the heavily damaged Surfside Beach/Garden City area. Most parts of both communities were still without electricity, but then there were few residents to need it. Virtually every ocean-front home had been destroyed.

There was no way to get a direct live shot out from the area because it was so far from our main tower. But sending the signal to this portable relay station I was making, then beaming it to the main facility, just might work.

We would need to use our own electricity to power the live truck and all of its equipment. For that, my crew off in the dark-ened distance would rely upon the truck's generator. Though the show was still nearly twenty-four hours away, we were working into the night to establish our first-ever "double-hop" live location. As I had proved during Hugo itself, planning ahead makes all the difference in live television.

Despite hours of exhausting work on the top of that building, I still couldn't make the link-up work. Our sister station in Pennsylvania put a new antenna on an airplane to Myrtle Beach when we called for help. It wouldn't arrive until after ten o'clock that night. Still, I wanted to get the live shot before we all went to bed.

Bill Christian was now involved, and I climbed down from the freezing ledge of the Palace to meet him at the airport. The new antenna in hand, I headed back to the Palace, and Bill and the live truck drove off into the blowing darkness.

By the time the truck had reached its destination, I was back on the roof and had the new antenna installed. I remembered Dr. Cheney telling me that some CFS patients have trouble retaining their body temperature. I was so cold now that I could hardly push the transmit button on my portable radio, and when I did, my lips barely moved. I wrapped a sheet of clear plastic around my body to fight off the biting wind.

Bill radioed that he had the truck's microwave transmitter turned on and pointed in my direction. I had been through this drill dozens of times earlier in the evening with the flawed set-up. The live truck would swing its antenna in an arc that would hopefully hit my tiny receiver twenty miles away. I would know if I had a usable signal when the receiver's signal strength meter climbed above 20.

Staring into the darkness of Surfside Beach and Garden City, I remembered my impressions of them the morning after Hugo, and how I trod through mud, debris, raw sewage, and the remnants of people's lives, helping to gather the story in the days that followed the storm. This night, I looked down the blackened coastline, then clicked on my flashlight to watch the signal strength meter.

"Ready!" I managed to say into the two-way radio.

"Here goes," Bill replied. "Panning to the right . . ."

For a moment, nothing happened. Then, quite slowly, the sig-

nal strength meter rose from its peg. Five, ten . . . twelve . . . fifteen
. . . seventeen . . .

"That's it!" I radioed, as the meter hit the magic 20 and came
to a stop at around 26. Bill clicked the transmitter off and on so I
could verify that I was, indeed, seeing his signal on the meter.

"Bingo!" I shouted.

"That's a roger," Bill came back.

I surveyed the darkness again, where six months earlier there
had been thousands of lights, lives, and dreams, and where tonight
there was nothing at all.

Then I looked at the field strength meter one more time. Even
though I couldn't see it with my eyes, there was a signal out there.
Somewhere off in the distance, a small generator was powering a
portable microwave transmitter, and a five-foot antenna was beaming that signal toward me, atop a hotel in the far-off darkness.

It was just a spark, but there was no denying what my receiver
was telling me. There *was* life in Surfside Beach tonight. I managed a smile at the notion.

Another eighteen months would pass before my illness would
take my career away. Understandably, with the exception of what I
have written about here, I remember very little about the day-to-
day activities of that period. I was struggling to stay afloat, perhaps
struggling to stay alive, and I was losing the battle.

By the spring of 1992, two years after I stood atop the Palace, I was
still very sick. I rarely, if ever, left my home, except for the twice
weekly trips to Charlotte for my Ampligen. I was convinced that
whatever good the drug might be doing was being canceled by the
effort of traveling so far and so often.

That summer, Hettie and I made the decision to move to
Charlotte. She was offered a job at a school district in the area,
and within an hour we had a "For Sale" sign on our lawn. The
decision was a painful one, but in the end we came to terms with a
simple notion: Nothing was more important than my getting better—no house, no job, no hopes of ever returning to WPDE. In
one respect, I felt like a quitter leaving town, for I had never before
walked away from a battle. But in another, more positive sense, I

realized there was nothing "quitting" about what we were doing. We were really setting off to face the battle head-on.

We moved into our new home in Charlotte on September 14, 1992, firm in our resolve that we were doing the right thing. That same week, I appeared in a five-part CFS series on CNN. I didn't watch the series, even though the segments aired several times each day. I didn't want to see how bad I had looked back in June when the CNN crew had spent a morning with me in Florence. That was probably as ill as I had been since just before my diagnosis.

The day after we moved into our new home, I drove to Athens, Georgia to speak to a CFS support group. The appearance had been scheduled three months earlier, and we had no idea the date would coincide with my move or the CNN series. I was exhausted from the move, and by the time I arrived in Athens that evening, I was concerned that I might not be able to offer the encouraging, hopeful presentation I had planned. I wanted to update them on Ampligen and the other research, I wanted to tell them about what was happening in Charlotte and around the world to unravel the mystery of CFS, and I wanted to present myself as something of a victor over this foe. But I was weak and tired. I stopped in a parking lot just two blocks from where I was scheduled to appear and walked unsteadily around my car, trying to summon strength from somewhere.

The meeting room quickly filled beyond capacity, and I started to speak. We talked at first about the CNN series, since they had all been watching. In part one of the series, CNN showed video of me as a fit and trim weathercaster several years earlier, flying in an F-16 with the Thunderbirds, producing coverage of a professional tennis match, and reporting live from Hurricane Hugo. No one needed to tell me that I didn't look like the same person today.

I surveyed the group, wondering to myself how anyone in the world could enter that room and dismiss CFS as some sort of psychological illness. I saw pale and weakened bodies, heard stories of foreclosures and bankruptcies, and listened to a courageous group of people prop each other up as best they could.

Hope. I was there to offer hope, I reminded myself.

I told them my story, including how I believed an experimental drug had helped me for a while, could help me more, and could possibly help some of them one day. I passed around the empty bottle from my previous day's infusion, and, as I had in Butler, Pennsylvania, six months earlier, let them touch what they had only read about.

There was more to tell them. Since my health had bottomed out in June, I had begun a slight upward climb. I didn't tell them that I felt awful that night; I stuck to the big picture of what had been going on in my life.

And there was something else I was especially proud to share. Just two days earlier, for the first time in more than a year, I had appeared on TV in a role other than an interview subject in a CFS story. I was offered the chance to fill in as weathercaster on a Charlotte TV station on a Sunday morning, and I had done okay—not great, but okay. Still, I told them, it was a miracle that I would not have believed possible just a few months earlier. Their eyes lit up as I described the experience. It wasn't easy, and I had always believed that being a weathercaster was the easiest job in TV. I hardly made it through, in fact, and I got confused at one point, trying to explain the extended forecast. But I had made it, and yes, they would call me again sometime to fill in.

I forgot my exhaustion and got caught up in the excitement of the meeting. Most people facing difficult circumstances just want to know there is some hope, and my two-and-a-half minute weathercast the previous weekend had given them—and me—just that: Hope.

Maybe someday, I told them, we can all have important parts of our old lives back.

The meeting went longer than planned, and I didn't leave Athens until nearly ten o'clock. I had about a dozen offers to stay with people in Athens, but I was determined not to spend my second night as a new homeowner in a strange town. I made my way to Interstate 85, set the cruise control on my car, and concentrated on staying awake.

By the time I approached the outskirts of Charlotte, I was numb from exhaustion, and the lights of the city formed a blurred

image. I was as tired as I had been that night atop the Palace in
Myrtle Beach. I turned up the air conditioning to blow cold air
onto my face.

A half hour later, I climbed wearily into bed, thankful that I
had survived the drive and wondering if I had done any good in
Athens, and if Athens had done any good in me.

I replayed the meeting in my mind, and saw something in the
eyes of the people there. My own eyes were too tired to show much
of anything, but I know by the time the meeting had ended I saw
something in theirs.

It was hope.

Thinking back to that night in 1990 atop the Palace, surveying
the darkness caused by Hugo's devastation, I realized how very
much that night had in common with the night in Athens, the
people I met there, and the life I now live.

In the darkness, in the destruction, in the bitter cold emptiness
of a life turned on its side by a misunderstood illness, there can be,
there needs to be, there is reason for hope.

Peering into the darkness, I can see it now, and I want to share
it with others. My bright eyes may be dimmed, one eyelid may
droop, my smile may not be quite what it was, and sometimes I
may walk with unsteadiness and pain. But there is life in here, and
life is the first part of survival, and survival is the first part of
rebuilding.

Somewhere off in the unseen distance, there is a reason for
that hope, just as surely as I know Bill Christian was beaming a
fragile microwave signal to me from the flattened remains of
Surfside Beach on a cold and windy March night.

The hope may be only a spark, but it is enough to keep me
going.

24

HIDING THE HURT

Somewhere between that spark that keeps me going and the reluctant equilibrium you will read about in the next chapter, there is another component to this battle with CFS that I hardly ever talk about. It is just how very much I hurt, both physically and emotionally.

With that hurt comes an exhaustion in every fiber of my being, an aching for relief, a yearning for a normal life I want so much. Second prize, I suppose, would be having the world and the medical establishment better comprehend this disease, giving it the respect and attention it deserves, and working toward eliminating the incalculable suffering it visits upon so many people who are so much more sick than I.

I can't kid myself. None of that will come soon. And this misery certainly doesn't love company. It doesn't help me the least little bit to know there are untold thousands of people around the world enduring what I am enduring, living life one painful minute at a time.

The emotional hurt is what has haunted me from the start of this terrible process of loss, misunderstanding, and compromise.

One recent fall afternoon, lying in my bedroom trying to summon the strength to walk into the kitchen, I wondered to myself if anyone at all has any idea of how close I come at moments like this to just giving up. I first discussed this feeling with Dr. Robertson soon after my departure from TV, when life seemed to be spinning out of control. Even now, though, the temptation to simply end all this uphill fighting comes and goes regularly. At times my aching spirit is so very worn down that the escape route seems the only one worth traveling. This is not some abstract notion of suicide, as in when I would speed toward that narrow concrete bridge. This is a practical, "let's get it over with" thought. As they used to say in the introduction to the TV show *The Six Million Dollar Man*, "We have the technology." It is all there in my medicine drawer. I could do it in an instant. I give speeches to inspire others, I write what I can with a positive message, and I work daily to be an example of the good things that could happen to someone facing a serious chronic illness. But I hurt, inside and out, and I struggle daily with the notion of ending that hurt with my own selfish shortcut. To say otherwise would be a lie.

Garth Brooks's song "Much Too Young to Feel This Damn Old" tears me up when I hear it. When I hear those lyrics, I feel the aches that my optimistic exterior has hidden away, I lay open fears that are too scary to share with anyone else, I ponder the reality that *five years* have already gone by—five of what should have been the best years of my life.

The greatest of these emotions is the fear, something I rarely experienced until I noticed my memory and my strength slipping away. Now, fear is a constant, unwelcome companion. If I am in this condition in my early thirties, what will I be like in my forties, my fifties? Will I even *see* my forties?

There have been times in this experience when fear has washed over me like a wave breaking over a swimmer at the beach. It has knocked me down, kicked me around, and taken my breath away until I regain my footing, waiting for the next wave to hit.

When I first felt control of my life slipping away, the fear stared me straight in the eye. When the only career I knew was ripped from my grasp, fear was the spectator that saw it all. When my company's disability insurance carrier initially turned down my application for monthly benefits and I thought of losing everything Hettie and I had managed to scrape together in our marriage, fear was with me in the room when I put my face in my hands and wept the words I'll never forget, "I'm just about to give up, God. Please give me strength."

Fear was my roommate through several hospitalizations and

surgery. When all the morphine and Demerol and all the other drugs would not put me to sleep, fear stayed awake with me all night in the hospital room. What would tomorrow bring? If this is happening now, what will your future be like? How can you afford this? Is there yet something *else* wrong with you? Fear asks many questions, and most of them make me shudder.

Fear rode along in the ambulance that took me from my home one terrible spring morning in 1993. As I heard the doors of the ambulance slam closed with me inside, I was gripped by something much stronger than the straps that held me to the stretcher. It was a fear that this trip from our new home might well be my last. Later, when I was released from the hospital and Hettie helped me walk back into our house, I looked at the marks on our lawn made by the stretcher when they wheeled me away. Inside the house, the living room furniture had yet to be rearranged from the paramedics' hurried efforts to clear a path from my sickbed. If ever I considered myself immortal in the recklessness of my youth, that foolish notion was swept away then.

Fear of the AIDS test. Oh, how that scared me. Fear of multiple sclerosis. Fear of the results of hundreds of blood tests, liver enzymes, the MRI scan, and countless other investigations into the most minute parts of my body. Fear of what is going on in my brain. What *is* going on in my brain? I fear the answers as much as I fear the questions.

There is a loneliness, too, that comes even when I am surrounded by others. In the bellies of hospitals, where radiologists direct diagnostic procedures and the very ill are treated and monitored in the early morning hours, a loneliness creeps into the soul like an ache in the joints after a long journey. It does not go away quickly. Part of me has been forever changed by just being around that. Another part of me has been scared beyond my wildest imaginings by actually *being* a part of that.

I regret the days and nights alone, wasted. I regret not being able to be the husband I should be. I regret not being the son I should be, or the brother. Sometimes I regret not taking the time to be a parent, but having children would be foolish in my condition.

I regret the friends who have fallen by the wayside, and I regret pushing some of them out of my life in the early days of my illness. I wonder if they know why I did it. I regret lost income, promotions that didn't come, the good things that I never accomplished within my industry.

I have remorse for what could have been. The remorse and the loss I feel are nearly as strong as one might feel about a death. A very big part of me has died.

I look at Hettie, and I am humbled by her patience, her compassion, and her focused dedication to a man who bears the lame diagnosis chronic fatigue syndrome, and I feel guilt. Two types of guilt. The first is because I can only imagine the sacrifices she has endured, the hours in hospitals and physicians' waiting rooms, the emergency calls at work, the parts of her own life that have been put on hold and may never be regained, the things she can't have so that we can pay doctor and prescription bills. No wonder so many CFS patients see their marriages dissolve.

The guilt from the second source twists and stabs at my insides, demanding an answer. The question is a simple one, the answer must be, too: Would I, if our roles were reversed, be able to be all to Hettie that she is now to me? I suppose the very presence of guilt suggests I would not, though I pray I will never have to confront the answer to that question.

Another source of constant emotional pain for me is the hurt that comes from being misunderstood, from being called a liar, from not being believed. I have had doctors with diplomas and commendations covering their office walls tell me they don't believe in CFS. Case closed. Come live with me for a week, I want to say, but the hurt and the shame—yes, shame—keep me silent. I am ashamed of this diagnosis. I am ashamed to speak the words *chronic fatigue syndrome*. I am ashamed to hear them. They are impotent, reviled words to me. They do not describe the people I know who cannot lift their heads from their pillows or cannot help their children dress for school. Those words do not describe a former NFL football player and street-hardened cop I know who isn't able to attend a single moment of his son's Little League games.

Those words do not describe me. Something is very wrong with my body, and it is not just immense tiredness. I had been exceptionally healthy until I approached my thirtieth birthday, and something very bad happened. Something may have gone wrong in my brain, in my cells, in my immune system—maybe all three—but I did not simply get fatigued. Shame has stolen much of my dignity, and it will remain that way until this disease is renamed.

I have seen television news programs about the follies of the experimental drug process, and I have recalled how I rolled the dice for three years, not having the slightest notion what that concoction being pumped into my veins might be doing to my heart, my liver, my kidneys. I look at the scars on my hands from hundreds of IV needles and I wince more from the uncertainty, more from the dashed hopes, more from the cure that didn't cure, than I do from the pain of a needle stick. Even a thousand needle sticks.

Physical pain is with me at virtually every moment. Even if I were healthy in every other way, the pain would dog me, it would hunt me down, it would wear me out. CFS patients experience varying degrees and types of pain at different times. For me, it is most often my muscles and my joints that scream out at me, though I am at times nearly blinded by roaring headaches.

The muscle and joint pain are enough to shut my life down. If I walk more than a few dozen yards, the pain causes me to limp and eventually forces me to stop. If I'm on my feet much during a day, I must wrap my ankles in Ace bandages to keep them still at night or the pain would never let me sleep. Hundreds of times I have gotten up from bed and climbed into a scalding hot bath to seek some relief—any relief.

Even such a simple action as typing on my keyboard to write this is disrupted by pain. For weeks at a time, I've had to wrap my wrists in bandages to lessen the motion and reduce the pain. I've had to keep my thumb in a splint and retrain my typing motions.

Leg muscles cramp into tight knots and shake and twitch painfully every night. If I sit at my desk for more than a few minutes, the cramping muscles in my back often force me closer and closer to the desk until I am nearly doubled over.

There is pain in my head, too, most of the time, a pressure that seems inescapable and is described by virtually all CFS patients. My eyes burn when I read or watch television. My throat is nearly always inflamed.

And I am one of the lucky patients who is not confined to bed. There are many whose pain is so severe that they receive constant infusions of powerful medication usually reserved for cancer patients or others with terribly painful conditions. I do have pain medication, and I use it without shame when I need to. I used to have one of those "I can tough it out" attitudes about pain, but there is no macho solution to fighting this pain. It is bigger than I am. It can outlast my will. It can find me anywhere, anytime.

A document entered into my Social Security disability hearing told of a test that actually quantified my pain. "Severe, chronic, and intractable," are the only words I remember from that report. It does something to you when you see your pain documented by experts in those stark terms.

But I don't want strong drugs to numb my view of the world. I already see so much of it quite dimly. My eyes blur, my ears ring, I cannot smell a thing, my fingers and toes are often numb, and certain medications alter what sense of taste has survived. My dominant sense of the world is pain.

Pain is my sixth sense; at times it is my only sense.

I smile and I give pep talks to patients and even some medical professionals. "It will work out," I tell them all. "We'll get through this . . . we'll get well again. It *has* to happen!" I tell them all.

And when I am alone, I wonder if the optimism they see—the outlook on life that seems to get me through this all—might just be the most basic form of denial there is. Maybe, despite all that I know, see, and feel, I just won't face up to the reality of this terrible disease. I can't believe it will shatter another marriage, ruin another career, put someone else out on the street. I can't believe what the CDC is considering as it looks at redefining this illness in the near future, actually poised to define it out of existence. That just *can't* happen. I can't conceive of the proposed national health care system that opponents say could ravage people with chronic, hard-to-pinpoint ailments. Looking back on medical bills that easily top $100,000, I wonder what I would have done had that system been in place when I first became ill. What will I do tomorrow if that system is in place and I am sent only to the doctors the government says I can see? What if those doctors don't believe in this illness? What if they don't believe me? Can I take another terrible trip through the rejection and brutality of a disbelieving medical system?

I can't handle the notion that this thing could be contagious, that it could be growing, that it could be our next AIDS and we're doing so little as a nation to stop it. I can't accept that we haven't pinpointed a cause, let alone put forth a successful treatment or cure. I can't rationally consider all of that or I would be overwhelmed by the cumulative hopelessness. Instead, I exude optimism and keep the fear and concern to myself. That optimism is genuine, no matter what makes it happen, and the supply seems to be holding up. But just below the surface there is so much more. There is exhaustion of indescribable magnitude, fear, loneliness, regret, remorse, guilt, misunderstanding, shame, physical pain, and so much more. And even when I succeed in blocking all of that from my conscious thoughts, there is the one reminder that is with me with every step I take, every wish I have, every ambition I cherish, every compromise that takes another part of my life away: it is the constant emotional and physical hurt that never goes away.

There is so much I want to do. If you know nothing else about me, you know that I love life, every part of it. I love just seeing sunsets. I love traveling. Every Friday afternoon, it seems as if we should be loading the car or heading to the airport, off to Baltimore's Inner Harbor, Charleston's historic district, or the spectacular North Carolina mountains. I still want to show Hettie the view from Point Loma in San Diego and the shimmer of dusk in the hills around Los Angeles, both of which I experienced on business trips and promised to share with her someday. I want to go back to spring training and walk around the waterfront in St. Petersburg or Vero Beach before having a great seafood dinner.

I want to cross the water again in a single-engine plane, finding a tiny Bahamian island and squeezing onto its pint-sized landing strip. I want to go camping, I want to be able to visit my family in Pennsylvania, I want to order room service and read a wine list. I want to plan a trip *anywhere* and actually go through with it.

I want to be a manager again, delivering ratings and watching the bottom line for my company. I want to interview young job applicants starting out on their careers, I want to pick the cream of that crop and teach them excellence, I want to be the innovative broadcaster I used to be.

There are less-complicated things I want in my life. I'd like to go to the mall and just take my time, rather than knowing I've got about five minutes of energy before I start limping and reaching for a wall or handrail to steady my walk. I'd like to go out to dinner on a moment's notice, I'd like to watch a Charlotte Hornets basketball game from somewhere other than the sofa, I'd like to go to a movie without having to plan my entire weekend around the two-hour outing. I'd like to be able to balance my checkbook again. I would like to be able to *remember* again.

I'd like to mow the lawn, learn to be a carpenter like my grandfather, maybe even hang some wallpaper. And I want to run four miles and work out again until the sweat soaks my shirt and my heart races with the thrill of aerobic exhilaration. Oh, how I want to do that!

But I can't do any of this, and I don't know when—or if—I'll be able to do it again, no matter how optimistic I sound, no matter how upbeat my message, and it is all because of something foolishly dubbed chronic fatigue syndrome. Oh, that I were fatigued!

This is all a rare admission from me. There are CFS patients in every state, in small towns and in big cities, in hospitals and in bedrooms, whose wants are so much simpler and whose pain is so much greater. They only want something to cling to, their own spark of hope that things might improve sometime, that life might return to a shadow of what it once was.

I hurt when I think of those people and hear of their shattered lives and countless losses. I hurt when I allow myself to consider my own condition, my own fears, my own pain. Most of all, though, I just plain hurt. All the time.

I am much too young to feel this damn old.

25
RELUCTANT EQUILIBRIUM

It is Sunday, October 10, 1993 in Charlotte, North Carolina. A brisk cold front has swept through the Carolina piedmont, rapidly chasing a brilliant sunset from the autumn sky. Charcoal-gray clouds are hurriedly painting the premature dusk into a bone-chilling darkness, and the temperature drops five degrees each passing hour. At 11:00 tonight, I will explain this hasty arrival of fall weather to thousands of TV viewers, and then—for the second time in just over two years—I will say goodbye to another television station. This time, though, my departure marks something of a new beginning, not a terrible ending.

Just as fall has chiseled a foothold into the Carolinas tonight, I have somehow managed to carve a new place in the world for myself in the year since I've moved to Charlotte. It will not be here at WCNC-TV as I had hoped, but—like the cool air mass that has everyone talking this evening—I think that maybe, just maybe, I'll be sticking around for a while.

More than five years have passed since I felt the beginnings of a sore throat while heading to flight school in Vero Beach, Florida; three and a half years since I first met Dr. Paul Cheney and learned that there was a name for the illness that was tearing my health, my career, and my plans to pieces. Twenty-six months have already gone by since I left my job as news director at WPDE, and it has been just over a year since we moved to our new home in Charlotte.

Without question, 1993—the fifth year of being sick—was the

most difficult period of my illness, filled with an unrelenting series of health setbacks.

I was in the hospital four times, admitted twice on an emergency basis, taken there once by ambulance. I had surgery, encountered a constellation of new neurological symptoms, and spent another year of sleepless nights and pain-filled days trying to get well, with little or nothing to show for it.

Somehow during that same period, I'd managed to work part-time at WCNC-TV as a weekend weathercaster. The station is Charlotte's NBC affiliate and headquarters of NBC's News Channel service and the network's overnight news program, *Nightside*.

WCNC had many of the same characteristics of WPDE, and I thought a thousand times how it would be great place to be a news director. The station was filled with dedicated and talented people, yet it faced a seemingly insurmountable uphill battle for ratings. That's my kind of challenge—leading a great team to do the impossible. A thousand more times, I wondered if such a move were preordained somehow, and I might have been headed for the kind of happy ending usually seen in made-for-TV movies. "Formerly disabled news director makes comeback—leads Charlotte station to ratings parity," I imagined the broadcasting trade papers might read one day.

I had visited WCNC just before my move to Charlotte in the summer of 1992, because I'd heard they needed someone to anchor the weather segment the following Sunday morning. I felt up to the one-time-only task, and I went on the air that weekend for the first time since I'd become ill.

In early 1993, I was invited to work the Sunday morning shift on a regular basis. (Ironically, I began my broadcasting career working Sunday mornings at a small AM radio station sixteen years earlier.)

The two-hour job each week paid enough to cover my monthly health insurance premiums. And being back inside a television station, if only for a couple of hours at a time, boosted my self-image. I had to miss work a few times because I was too sick or was in the hospital, but each time Larry Sprinkle—one of Charlotte's top television personalities and now the head weathercaster at WCNC—cheerfully covered for me.

Several months after I had taken over the Sunday morning shift, a change in the station's anchor team created an opening for another weekend weathercaster—one who could work both Saturdays and Sundays, mornings and evenings. For several days, I wondered if I had the endurance to work two days a week, a couple of hours at a time. I wasn't sure of the answer, but I spoke up and asked the news director to consider me for the job.

With apologies to my many friends who are weathercasters and meteorologists, I should explain that the actual on-air part of being a weathercaster is one of the least-taxing jobs in the universe, providing you have been blessed with the ability to string coherent sentences together without a lot of "ums" thrown in. You must also be able to point to a blank wall in roughly the same spot as the weather features you are describing, while looking into a television monitor at a reverse image of yourself superimposed over computer-generated maps. And, of course, you need to know something about the weather and be able to explain it in everyday terms while a producer talks into your earpiece. Plus, you need to be able to do all this in *exactly* the time the producer allots you, which he or she often decides to change partway through your presentation.

Okay, so maybe it's not easy, but I had reason to believe I could do it.

I've never been short on words, so the first part of the job would be no problem. Give me a microphone, and I'll talk forever.

The second requirement for the job was easy for me as well. I could look into a monitor where east was west and west was east and still manage to point my index finger somewhere in the vicinity of where I wanted it to be, just as naturally as some people knot their ties without being able to explain exactly how they do it.

My aviation training and experience had given me an excellent practical understanding of weather dynamics, so I considered myself qualified for that part of the job, too. The only remaining issue was my health. When I was in charge of WPDE's news department, I had actually demoted myself from the job of backup weathercaster because I wasn't dependable once I'd gotten sick.

The question dogging me now—just months after surgery and a few weeks after my most recent hospitalization—was again one of reliability: Could I push my fragile endurance and work two days every week, even though the actual physical task would be relatively easy?

Unsure of the answer and hoping that fate would decide for me, I kept asking for the job, and the answer kept being "no."

The station management told me they would be hiring someone else for the job—someone "more qualified," I was told by the news director. But he did ask if I could anchor most of the weekend weathercasts on a temporary basis until someone else was hired.

I was insulted and hurt to know that I wasn't being considered for the new position, but my eagerness to work at something I felt I could do outweighed my injured pride. For several weeks, therefore, I agreed to be the primary weekend weathercaster at WCNC, while the search for another candidate went on.

Although the job was not physically taxing, the effort required to be *anywhere* on a consistent basis immediately began taking a heavy toll on me. For those weeks that I appeared cheerful and upbeat in three-minute weekend weather segments, I did nothing else anywhere. I spent most of my time in bed, searching for rest and energy that eluded me, emerging in a jacket and tie on Saturdays and Sundays as a television personality. It was a senseless barter of what little energy I had for a few minutes of being part of a TV news team, but I made the trade eagerly, anxious to have something to show for my life again. Against every bit of good judgment I had, I asked WCNC's news director several more times if he would consider moving me permanently into the position, and his answer—thankfully—remained the same. The search for my replacement would go on.

Knowing my time at the TV station was coming to an end, I wrestled with the notion of losing my professional identity again, the notion of becoming a "disabled former broadcaster" for a second time. Hettie and the few friends that honestly knew about my situation urged me to leave the weekend weather job even before a permanent replacement was found. But, just as in my final days before leaving WPDE, I refused to listen to reason. I continued to work weekends at WCNC, all the while seeing myself sink deeper into the permanent exhaustion and unrelenting weakness of CFS.

Just a few weeks after I took on the extra weathercasting duty, WCNC's three top news management positions became available: news director, assistant news director, and special projects producer. The notion that these jobs were open and I didn't have the strength to do any of them dealt me a hard psychological blow. Since moving to Charlotte, I had been convinced that there would someday be a place for me at WCNC.

Then, one morning I came across an idea that changed my life. I was beginning to experience mixed emotions knowing that my part-time job was ending when I stumbled upon a job that seemed like something I might be able to do. Maybe there really *was* a way to work again, using my experience and talents as a broadcaster without the terrible tradeoff I was experiencing from the weather position. The idea popped up faster than an afternoon thunderstorm in the Carolinas, and I moved on it immediately.

I approached Ron Ellis, the program director at WTDR-FM, one of Charlotte's leading radio stations, and asked about becoming his traffic reporter. WTDR was using an outside service that provided traffic information to several Charlotte stations in exchange for commercial spots. I asked Ron to consider hiring me as WTDR's own traffic reporter, a potentially beneficial move for the station if I could compete with the service being offered by other stations in town, and a job that would require only light physical exertion. Little did I know that WTDR had been contemplating making such a move for several months—if only it could find the right person for the position. There was yet another consideration the station was facing, too, and this one had my name written all over it.

WTDR's parent company had just purchased a second station in the Charlotte market—WEZC-FM—and its program director, Mike Berlack, was interested in sharing the new traffic reporter with WTDR. But the acquisition of WEZC meant the two stations would be located in the same office building, and space would be at a premium. Where would the traffic reporter work? Ron and Mike explained that they hadn't designated a location as a traffic information center in the new facility. The telephones, computers, police radios, emergency service scanners, audio processors, and other equipment necessary for the job would take up an entire studio or office, so the traffic reporter would be forced to work from a remote location. That was the opening I'd been hoping for.

When Hettie and I first looked at the plans for our new home in Charlotte a year earlier, we'd set one room aside as "Tim's office." For a year, it had contained only my writing desk and a computer, along with some memorabilia from my broadcasting career. With some modifications to that office, I could provide WTDR and WEZC the extra studio and traffic information center the stations needed, and I could finally make a return to full-time broadcast news reporting right from my home. The new studio and office would be electronically linked to the WTDR and WEZC studios, providing the stations' listeners with a state-of-the-art information source, while providing me a new career that seemed likely to be within my capabilities.

After a few weeks of discussions, WTDR and WEZC made me a generous offer, and I eagerly accepted the job as their new traffic reporter. We reached our agreement exactly two years to the day that I'd left WPDE dejected and broken, convinced that my broadcasting career was over. Maybe it wasn't "Movie of the Week" material, and maybe I wasn't yet healthy, but the word *miracle* began to make a regular appearance in my vocabulary.

On that chilly evening of October 10, waiting to do my last weathercast at WCNC, I walked alone through the high-tech facility in a sort of silent farewell and thank-you. This station in the twenty-ninth-largest TV market was a long way from the smaller WPDE in Florence/Myrtle Beach, South Carolina, but the two operations had much in common. At each, I had carved out a professional identity and a sense of worth and self-esteem I needed desperately and hadn't possessed before. As I had in the Florence/Myrtle Beach market, I'd made a few friends in Charlotte, too, and at a time when friendships were at a premium, I was sorry to be leaving. But my new radio job left no room for compromise. Even though my traffic office was just down the hall from my living room, I would need 100 percent of my strength and ability to keep the commitment I'd made to it.

As I had when I'd left WPDE, I carefully committed to memory the sensations of my final hours at WCNC. Just before air time, I sat alone in the weather center and quietly gave thanks for the three-minute miracles that had taken place there. A short time later, I went on TV for the last time.

After that 11:00 news broadcast, I shook hands with my weekend co-workers, feeling my throat beginning to tighten as I said goodbye. Then, I slipped back to the solitude of the weather center, only the hum of computers breaking the silent spell of that small room. Save for my writing desk at home, this was the only place in the world where I'd had a sense of professional belonging and identity over the past two years.

With a personal introspection and self-searching contemplation that not even CFS and my brain injury could take away from me, I spent those private minutes trying to recall the past year since I'd moved to Charlotte, and all that had led to this moment.

I was still sick, still in the grips of a mysterious and misunderstood disease. The CFS "recovery" that I'd read about in popular magazines had not happened to me, nor had it happened to any of the other patients I knew. Little by little, though, I realized that I had recovered some of the pieces of my life that meant the most to me, despite this terrible illness. From time to time—for maybe an hour or so—windows of wellness and function would open, and I could go out to lunch or dinner, or go with Hettie when she went shopping. I had even been to a few movies, traveled to Ohio to see my friend Tom Sorrells get married, and hired an instructor to let me play around in a small airplane. In lieu of a recovery of my health, these tiny windows—and the life-bits I recovered during them—were a welcome consolation prize. Although the windows closed as quickly as they opened, they did offer me hope for the future.

Also, over the past year, the Ampligen drug trial had finally and abruptly ended amidst more confusion and unanswered questions. There was no indication whether the experimental drug had proved to be effective over the long term. No one could tell me when or if I might get it again, and no one had yet been able to tell me if a thousand IV needles and moving to Charlotte had made even the slightest difference to my shattered immune system. The FDA had refused to approve the drug at that point, and I left Ampligen with its future very much in question.

Despite all these questions and real concerns about not receiving the drug, there was a good part to ending my involvement with Ampligen. I no longer faced the IV needles and physical side effects I attributed to the infusions, and I no longer needed to expend precious energy going to the doctor's office twice each week.

Another memory of the past year was a trip to Washington, D.C. Along with several other CFS patients and advocates, I'd gone there shortly after President Clinton's election, invited to attend meetings with his health care transition team, one voice among millions trying to get the attention of a new administration. I'd also traveled to Orlando, where I had the pleasure of speaking to the Central Florida CFS Support Group, of sharing my story, of the group's members sharing their warmth.

Nearly two years after my initial application for Social Security disability, I'd finally gotten a hearing before an administrative law judge. The hearing actually came two weeks after I accepted my new radio traffic job, but the judge believed me, and that's what I had been fighting for.

And, just three weeks before my final weathercast at WCNC, I was asked to fill in as executive producer of the 5:30 and 6:00 newscasts for a few days. That meant—for four hours a day for one week in September—I was once again working at the top of a television news department. Like my ride in the F-16 just before I quit flying several years earlier, the experience was a reinforcement of my dignity and determination—one very special glimpse at the peak before settling into a life filled with compromise.

Compromise. I thought about that word in those moments I sat alone in the WCNC weather center after my final TV appearance. Was that really what I was doing now, or was something much more dramatic taking place in my life?

I remembered the words of Liz Crosby, Diversified Communications' human resources manager, when I'd called her to discuss leaving the company back in August 1991.

"Maybe this is your second chance . . . maybe you'll get through this," she said after I explained my illness and my need to leave. "Maybe you'll be back someday."

My second chance. This was it.

There was no compromising as I left TV broadcasting this time. I was leaving for my second chance, my new career. This was a victory in my redefined life, not a compromise. It might not be the same as dodging hurricanes, but I knew I could get good, timely traffic information on the air and help thousands of people, and I knew I could still make the competition sit up and take notice.

I spent a few moments there in the weather center thinking about the other CFS patients I know across the country who have yet to get their second chances, and I thought of those who never will. I thought about people with multiple sclerosis, AIDS, cancer, and all those things that don't ever make room for a second chance.

I don't know why things happen as they do. I don't know why it's me this time and not them. I don't know why, in the midst of all that CFS has visited upon me, I have been able to find little windows of life that offer glimpses of a more complete and perhaps total recovery that might really come someday.

As I prepared to leave WCNC for the last time, I wondered if there might be a phrase to describe the new life that I had to live now—that I was lucky enough to live now—this second chance Liz and a few others had said might come my way. There had to be a simple yet positive way to describe the parameters within which I would now exist. As a writer and reporter, I used to be able to condense anything into a few words, and I felt the need to do that now before I let the door close on my TV career one last time. I needed something to call this last chapter of my struggle for recovery, something to remind me of what I had to do to make this work.

Alone in a hallway leading to WCNC's parking lot, I paused for a moment, searching my mind for the right phrase. It was slow in coming, because words still do not occur to me as quickly as they once did.

I didn't want to leave the TV station that night until I found that phrase, because leaving television now meant accepting a new way of life and a new future, and I needed a way to describe that process. I know that when the door to WCNC closed behind me, I would be exchanging the unrealistic dream of returning to television for a realistic but downsized new way of life—a way of life that I thought could be successful. I needed a way to describe this new life that was nothing like my old life, words that would depict the careful balance I was seeking between compromise and victory.

"Reluctant equilibrium" came to mind.

I repeated the phrase in my mind a few times, satisfied that it would do just fine.

Promising myself I would strive to maintain this reluctant equilibrium and maximize my life's second chance no matter what might happen, I scribbled the phrase onto a scrap of paper and stepped out into the brisk October night.

I glanced at the impressive television facility one last time in my car's mirror, saying farewell to the dreams and hopes that had once meant so much to me. It didn't hurt nearly as much this time around, and I think I know why.

At some time between leaving the television studio and cranking my car's engine, the reluctance I had just defined gave way to something else, something more akin to my character. It was a cautious sense of optimism. I rode home that night buoyed by a new sense of eagerness, and driven by an even greater determination to beat this thing called chronic fatigue syndrome.

EPILOGUE
A Spouse's Tale

For as long as I can remember, I've wanted to teach exceptional children. When I finished college in 1982, I began working as an elementary school speech pathologist. I moved into a position working with hearing-impaired students, and most recently I have taken over what is called a cross-categorical classroom. When people ask me what I do, I go into an awkward explanation of how I teach a group of primary-aged students with a variety of handicaps. Invariably, my listener comments on how patient I must be to work with such students. No, I quickly point out, patience isn't the important element—I love what I do.

A similar formula has helped me survive the challenge and demands of Tim's illness. It takes more than patience when you're married to a chronically ill person. I've learned to be flexible, yet firm. I find ways to love what I do.

Love has become a verb, not a passive feeling. I listen, talk, pick up the slack, carry on, make do. I find myself doing a myriad of things I've never done before and really didn't expect to do at this point in my life: following ambulances, completing endless insurance forms, talking with each new doctor or technician after each new procedure. I now slip effortlessly into medical jargon in my everyday speech. As if this onslaught of changes were not enough, I find so little time to stop and think. My life's routines—now hopelessly splintered—still go on, though compounded by the need to be more than what I've ever had to be in the past.

Through it all, I've managed to carve out a sense of cautious optimism. I honestly feel things will work out. But I'm also a realist—things won't work out tomorrow.

Tim's chronic illness is with me every moment. My husband

has physical and cognitive disorders that require understanding and compassion, but his is a disease that is misunderstood by the general public and not recognized by many physicians. In the midst of medical crises, I frequently have to make difficult decisions with little or no guidance from the medical establishment.

I was not always so pragmatic. After Tim was first diagnosed, I was convinced he would soon die and I would be alone, a very young widow. I played his funeral over and over in my head. I saw my life crumbling all around me. I knew I could never live a happy and full life without Tim.

Within six months, I was on the verge of a personal crisis of my own, trying to cope with his illness and his needs, while trying to adjust to my own feelings. I had little support. No one I knew really understood the disease. Some friends were kind enough to listen, but they could offer little help. Adjusting to the external changes in my life was a matter of scheduling and stamina, but the internal things—the thoughts, fears, and doubts that ran unchecked through my mind—tormented me. What did our future hold? Would our marriage be ruined? Would Tim become bedridden and completely dependent on me? Could our finances stand the strain? Would we have to sell the house? Could anything good be made out of this? My feelings were in a jumble, and I didn't know how to verbalize them in a meaningful way.

Fortunately, I found a professional counselor who helped me express myself in a safe environment. In time, she taught me that what I was feeling was entirely normal, and I took some measure of comfort from that realization.

I can now say that the early days after Tim's diagnosis was a time of great personal growth for me, but at that time all I recognized was the pain. For weeks I walked around in a haze. I did my job and took care of things around the house, but I did nothing else. I was devastated. As an itinerant teacher, I traveled to schools over a five-county area. Being alone in my car for hours a day gave my fears and feelings plenty of time to confront me, and many times I cried so hard I could hardly see the road. The world as I'd known it was slipping away. Tim was just trying to survive each day. He didn't want to talk specifically about his symptoms, and he no longer wanted to talk about his day at work. His energy went into his job and his denial.

Through counseling, I realized that I needed to discuss my feelings meaningfully with Tim. Ordinarily, I would bottle my feelings up inside and periodically blow up at Tim. There was no in-between. I learned to operate somewhere in the middle, to voice my opinion without exploding.

Bit by bit, I began to speak openly with Tim. It was difficult and at first I wasn't very good at it, but I knew it was necessary. Tim needed to understand that his illness affected both of us. If I hadn't gotten help and learned to talk with Tim frankly about my thoughts and feelings, I don't think our marriage would have survived those first terrible months of adjustment.

Today, the adjustment continues, and I feel our marriage is better than it was before Tim got sick. Always good friends, Tim and I have developed a bond forged by crisis and strengthened by the triumph of survival. But as with everything else that we have to show for this experience, that bond did not come easily. In my mind, I can vividly see the turning point of our relationship back in 1991.

Tim, though very sick, was still working. He was in deep denial and was futilely trying to hold everything together. After one particularly difficult day for us both, we had a disagreement of major proportions. The blow-up had been brewing for several days and—as usual—it stemmed from his unyielding determination to devote all of his time and energy to the demands of his staff. As our dispute reached its boiling point, we both said things we would regret, and then Tim raised the stakes. He said he was leaving. He said it in such a way that I knew he meant it.

Shocked, I turned to Tim and told him, through my tears, that I wanted to be married to him forever, and that one day I wanted Paul Harvey to announce our wedding anniversary. I believe today that so much was accomplished with that one statement. More than taking on chores he could no longer do, more than being consumed by medical issues, more than trying to understand that his world, too, was slipping away, that statement told Tim that I had taken our marriage vows seriously and I *was* going to be with him through sickness and health. Our confrontation was diffused, but I knew the details needed to be worked out. That would take time, but it was a goal that from that day forward we undertook together, not separately.

I've proved over and over to Tim that I want to be his wife forever. I have done things for and with him that have amazed us both. From the very beginning, I went with him to doctor appointments, taking time off from work and driving him when he was too ill. I went with him to so many procedures: lumbar punctures, emergency room trips, blood tests, MRIs. I've spent hundreds of hours outside examination rooms, outside operating rooms, waiting. I've tracked down special prescriptions and talked with pharmacists about new drugs. When the situation became most difficult, I was there not because I had to be, but because I wanted to be—for Tim. I believe that often the right thing to do is the most difficult, and I have come to learn that there is very little glamor—but very great satisfaction—in fulfilling my commitment to my husband.

It is only with the gift of time that I can focus and draw conclusions about the past few years. When Tim first became ill, and even after the diagnosis, I never thought, "He's in denial," or "He's angry at the world." In the midst of all the confusion and changes, I couldn't see what was really happening, but I think I can see that now.

Tim doesn't take "no" for an answer—he is very stubborn. This is why he is working today; maybe it is why he is even around today. He must often take small steps to achieve a goal, but he almost always reaches that goal. I admire his strong will, but it can be difficult being on the other side of that powerful force.

In the early months of his illness, Tim's effort to maintain a regular work schedule took every bit of his energy. He would rise in the mornings having gotten virtually no sleep, and would painfully make his way into the office. He worked a full day, sometimes not getting home until 7:30. Then he would collapse. Sometimes, I had to help him from the car to the front door, and most days he never made it past the living room sofa. He couldn't read a book or even watch television. I had to screen his calls because his ability to talk was so limited.

I couldn't help but feel cheated, thinking that the TV station was getting Tim's best, leaving me with the leftovers. It was vitally important to Tim that he continue working. I understood that, but it still frustrated me. Tim crashed each night, and I diligently tried to hold everything together. It was a sad time that seemed to go on forever. Tim was so sick, and he was getting worse. We were both terribly strained by the situation, even though we were trying to pull together.

I could not truly comprehend how Tim was feeling. I tried to be empathetic, but I did not understand why he wouldn't take some time off work—even just a day. It seemed to me that if he could catch up on his rest and sleep, that he might begin to feel just a little bit better. But he never took a day off; his will to "proceed as normal" was too strong. Fortunately, there came a day when Tim recognized that leaving his job was inevitable. That was another turning point, which brought its own daily challenges and difficulties.

Those first few months after Tim left WPDE reminded me of an experience from nearly a decade earlier. We had just brought home a new puppy, a Cairn terrier we named Lexie. Sometimes he was a terror. When we came home we'd open the door fearfully, uncertain of what we'd find. Puddles and chewed socks, ruined shoes and pillows, house plants systematically destroyed and potting soil spread everywhere. It still confounds us that he once actually unzipped a sofa cushion and then removed the pillow and shredded it, leaving the cover perfectly intact. However, there were other times that we'd return home to find our sweet little puppy curled up in a ball, dozing quietly, the house in perfect order.

When Tim had to quit work, I experienced similar feelings on a much more serious level. I would call him several times during the day to check on him. It was important for me to know how he was feeling, physically and emotionally. He had suffered such a deep loss, I was afraid to think of what he might do. I also wanted him to know that I was thinking of him, that he wasn't alone. And

I always called just before I left work; as much as anything, I needed to prepare myself for what I might find when I got home.

Tim's mood would range from miserable to amiable, and it sometimes changed during my brief ride home. I knew that he had no control over these swings—his body was a war zone. He was dealing with issues physically and mentally: his days were empty and he was so frustrated. Understanding all of that, however, did not make the experience any easier.

Tim's body is still a war zone and how he feels continues to fluctuate. He tends to cycle in good and bad phases, but within each phase are periods of functioning contrasted with times of virtual immobility. Even at his best times in the good cycles, he never feels like a healthy person. He is always limited, always hurting, always fighting.

It is impossible to predict how well or poorly Tim will be feeling on a given day. How he was feeling the night before or even that very morning is no indicator of how his day will be. One morning in spring 1993, for example, I slipped out of the house because Tim appeared to be sleeping quite deeply. Several hours later, he was being rushed to the hospital in an ambulance, and I was trailing behind in my car. He hadn't been sleeping: he'd had a severe reaction to some new medication and was slipping in and out of consciousness.

Because of the unpredictable nature of his health, any plans we make are tentative. We have canceled so many things we had planned to do that I no longer keep count. Trips to visit family and friends, vacations, dinner out, movies—even trips to the supermarket—have all fallen into a pile of things stolen by CFS. I don't blame Tim; like he has done, I've learned to blame this illness. This is just how things are at this point in our lives, and I live with the knowledge that it might be this way forever. I also live with the knowledge that this is, at least, better than not being together at all.

When Tim first began to cancel things we had planned, I became frustrated and angry, especially before we knew what was wrong with him. I felt as if life was passing us by, and I didn't know why. That frustration and anger is understandable. We were supposedly in the prime of our lives. We finally had some financial stability, and we were supposed to be out enjoying life. Friends and co-workers were always going places and doing things. It was our time to have some fun.

The first major plans we canceled were in early 1989, a year before Tim was diagnosed. His cousin, Carol, and her family live near Washington, D.C., and we planned a trip to visit them and to tour the capital. Everything was arranged. I had packed our bags, and our hosts were expecting us.

Then Tim called me from work and said he couldn't make the trip because he just wasn't up to it. I couldn't believe it. It was so maddening. We were packed—all we had to do was get in the car and go, but for some reason, Tim said he didn't have the strength and energy for the short trip. Privately I thought that once again the station was getting Tim's best, leaving me with nothing. Since then, of course, I have seen events much less demanding than a weekend trip scrubbed all the time, and we have somehow learned to adjust.

I can never fully count on our best intentions to go anywhere, even to the video store to rent a movie. Tim's health has remained far too variable to depend upon, but I deal with that differently now. We might cancel something we have planned, there is no such thing for us as making "simple" plans, but we have each other and we have the future. Maybe we missed the Christmas tree lighting or Fourth of July fireworks, but we have learned simply to enjoy the time we spend together. I try to focus on what I have, not on what I've missed. I am still disappointed at times, but by focusing toward the positive and away from the negative, I don't waste valuable time and energy.

The process of coping with the new parameters of life continues to evolve. In my training as a teacher of children with special needs, I have been taught to look for areas of weakness and adapt the environment to meet those needs. If a child can't write with a pencil, maybe he can type at a computer. If a student can't talk, I train her in sign language or in using picture boards to communicate. If he is impulsive, I teach him control.

This concept carries over into my whole life. I am constantly trying to adapt the environment to help Tim. If he can't eat dinner at the table, I take him a tray in bed. If he is frustrated or having neurological difficulties, I eliminate the distractions of dogs, telephone calls, even background noises. If his pain becomes too intense for him to bear, I get his medication or massage his muscles.

I've tried to become familiar with the process of CFS so I can comprehend what is happening, why it is happening, and what to do about it. Learning about any major disability or illness leads to better understanding of its impact. CFS is complicated, poorly defined, and difficult to treat, and its symptoms wax and wane. By learning all I can about the disease, I can more easily be supportive to Tim and adapt to the limitations CFS brings to him.

Perhaps what I have missed most of all in this experience has been talking to other people like me, other spouses with a sick partner. I'm not sure why I didn't seek out someone else in my situation when this all first began, but I wish that I had. I've always been hesitant to speak openly about my feelings, and initially I wasn't even sure what those feelings were. But even if I had wanted to meet other people in my situation, I don't know where I would have turned to do so. In 1990, there were no CFS support groups listed in the Sunday papers, there were no books about how to cope with this disease or how to deal with what all I was in for, there was no one for me to lean on and learn from.

In the months after his diagnosis, Tim frequently talked to other CFS patients by phone or computer, and the time spent receiving his Ampligen infusions turned into mini-support group meetings. Though he now prefers not to talk about CFS much with patients or anyone else, I think at that time he found comfort in knowing he was not alone in his struggle. I now wish that I had looked for someone who was in the same situation as I; I'm sure it would have helped us both.

Like many wives, I find my role has changed over the years of our marriage. Back when I got married—I was 18—I certainly didn't anticipate that I would be in this situation. I just wanted to spend time with the man I loved. But even back then I had a sense of the commitment it would take to make a marriage survive, and that sense has served me well during this time.

In the early years of our marriage, Tim and I shared the responsibilities of managing our household. He paid the bills, I washed dishes, we both did the laundry. It was actually fun to be our own family, and to do it as a team. We had a nice time growing up together.

Tim supported me as I finished college, and we moved to South Carolina a few moths after I graduated. We both found work that challenged and fulfilled us, and not long after that we bought our first home.

As Tim's work responsibilities grew, so did mine. I began to tutor a few students in the evenings, and I also took a part-time job in the state's home-based parent-infant program—all on top of my full-time teaching career. Our lives were busy, but we were happy.

Tim's job at the television station became increasingly demanding well before he became ill. He put in long days—even on weekends—and he often spent hours on the phone at night. Some of the household duties naturally shifted to me because I had more time, but Tim insisted on sharing as much of the load as his schedule would allow.

Eventually, though, as his illness took away so many of his abilities and so much of his strength, Tim asked me to do more and more. When he wasn't able to keep our bills paid on time, I took over that job, too. This was a huge milestone, for it was the one job Tim didn't want to relinquish. Admitting that he could no longer even make sense of the checkbook was frightening, for Tim had always been exceptional with math. Even that was being taken away. Eventually, I came to take on all of our household tasks, even overseeing the yard man we hired to keep our lawn.

I quit tutoring so I could spend more time at home. It was a difficult time for him and for me. We put dreams on hold. We changed our focus from the future to the present. Living day-to-day—sometimes hour-to-hour—became necessary and routine. We rarely spoke of the future because it represented a frightening unknown.

Several months after Tim left his job, when Tim was desperately ill, a friend asked a poignant question. "Do you at least have hope?" she queried cautiously. At that point, I'd lost virtually all of mine. Year after year of declining health with no measurable improvement is almost unbearable, and my hope was being replaced by fear and frustration. It was not until Tim began to show minor progress after we moved to Charlotte that my hope slowly began to return.

In times of crisis, people often turn either toward or away from religion. While this experience has tested me and stretched the limits of virtually every aspect of my life, it has not shaken my faith. Even during the period in which I had no real hope for the future, I still clung to my faith. The Bible teaches that hope and faith are closely related, yet I had lost hope for a while although I had not lost my faith.

Is that a contradiction? Did God make my husband sick? Was He responsible for all of this? Those are legitimate questions, and I have not considered them lightly.

I do not believe that God made Tim sick, nor do I believe that He is responsible for all the trials we have been through. Living as we do in the natural world, people sometimes get sick. But that was no reason for me to turn my back on my faith or to reject my belief in God.

Friends, co-workers, family members, and doctors have all disappointed me during this time, but God never has. At times, He has been the only source of comfort I have had. I have had doubts about the future and have questioned Tim's lack of progress, but I have not questioned God. He has helped me through this period. He meets me at my level—all I need to do is ask, and His comfort is there.

The Book of Hebrews asserts that faith is the substance of things hoped for, the evidence of things not seen. During the time when I could not hope—let alone see—a brighter tomorrow, my faith sustained me when my intellect and my own imagination could not.

That faith has proved worthy. Today, more than five years after

Tim first became ill, we are beginning to see a tiny pinpoint of light at the end of this tunnel.

Tim's strong will persists, and he continues to push himself to do more and more. I still take care of a majority of our household tasks, but Tim contributes more than he has in years. We are still trying to find the balance in our roles. There are still many days Tim can do very little, but thankfully, some days he can do quite a bit. He has created a job that is within his capabilities, despite being finally declared totally disabled by the Social Security Administration and eligible for full benefits if he wanted them.

At this point, Tim's biggest physical obstacle is pain—he is never without it. Never. Recently he had an evaluation called a pain map. This is a new, highly technical way to objectively quantify pain using sophisticated electronic monitors. The test concluded that Tim suffers chronic, intractable pain. There was concrete evidence of this in every category the test measured.

While there are many medications available to suppress the pain, the side-effects are often not only unpleasant, but disabling and potentially fatal. Tim has developed serious ulcers as a result of the medications, and he's had other problems too, including the severe reaction I mentioned earlier. There is also the possibility of dependency.

Tim has gradually stepped down from some of the strongest medication available to some of the mildest. Because his severe pain has been so dramatically documented, he could have the stronger medication any time he wanted it, but he chooses not to. Watching him hurt makes me hurt. It is terrible knowing your loved one is in tremendous pain.

Today, as Tim deals with his pain, works at his job, and continues to seek the latest medical developments and treatments, I find that the emotional aspects of having a sick husband are far more difficult to deal with than the practical ones. I have learned to be flexible and tolerant, and willing to do what needs to be done. It's what I promised to do when I married Tim, and it's what I will do forever.

* * *

When people learn of Tim's health situation and they see the demands it places on me, they comment on how hard this must be, and that I must be extremely patient. Patience is a practical part of it, I'm sure, just like it is a part of what I do in my classroom, but that's not what sustains me. What keeps me going more than anything else is that I truly love what I do.

A GUIDE TO CFIDS
CFIDS Association of America

What Is CFIDS? CFIDS (chronic fatigue and immune dysfunction syndrome) is also known as CFS (chronic fatigue syndrome), CEBV (chronic Epstein-Barr virus), ME (myalgic encephalomyelitis), "yuppie flu," and many other names. It is a complex illness characterized by incapacitating fatigue (experienced as exhaustion and extremely poor stamina), neurological problems, and a constellation of symptoms that can resemble other disorders, including mononucleosis, multiple sclerosis, fibromyalgia, AIDS-related complex (ARC), Lyme disease, post-polio syndrome, and autoimmune diseases such as lupus. These symptoms tend to wax and wane but are often severely debilitating and may last for many months or years. All segments of the population (including children) are at risk, but women under the age of forty-five seem to be the most susceptible.

What Causes CFIDS? Research suggests that CFIDS results from a dysfunction of the immune system. The exact nature of this dysfunction is not yet well defined, but it can generally be viewed as an up-regulated or overactive state (which is responsible for many of the symptoms). Ironically, there is also evidence of some immune suppression in CFIDS; patients exhibit certain down-regulated signs. For example, in many patients there are functional deficiencies in natural killer cells (an important component of the immune system responsible for protection against viruses).

Based on physical and laboratory findings, many scientists are convinced that viruses are associated with CFIDS and may be directly involved in causing the disease. Since the discovery (or rediscovery) of CFIDS in the United States in the mid-1980s, several viruses have been—and continue to be—studied to determine what, if any, part they play in the disease. These include enteroviruses, herpesviruses (especially human herpesvirus-6 or HHV-6), and novel (newly discovered) retroviruses.

In the first few years of this research, it was thought that the Epstein-Barr virus (EBV), a herpesvirus that causes mononucleosis, was the cause of this syndrome. However, researchers now believe that EBV activation (when it exists) is a result or complication of CFIDS rather than its cause. To date, no virus has been conclusively shown to be an essential element of CFIDS.

Accordingly, research efforts are still directed toward identifying and isolating the fundamental agent(s) responsible for triggering immune system disruption in persons with CFIDS (PWCs). Additionally, there are ongoing studies of immunologic, neurologic, and metabolic abnormalities and co-factors (such as genetic predisposition, age, sex, prior illness, other viruses, environment, and stress) which appear to play an important role in the development and course of the illness. For further information, see the *CFIDS Chronicle*, which reports extensively on all aspects of CFIDS research, or call the CFIDS Information Line (900-896-2343) for the most recent developments in CFIDS research.

How Is CFIDS Diagnosed? Many physicians base their diagnosis of CFIDS on a "working case definition" developed by the Centers for Disease Control (CDC) and published in the March 1988 *Annals of Internal Medicine*. To meet the CDC case definition, a patient must fulfill two "major criteria" *and* either eight of eleven "symptom criteria" or six of the symptom criteria *and* two of three "physical criteria."

The major criteria are as follows: (1) "New onset of persistent or relapsing, debilitating fatigue or easy fatigability in a person who has no previous history of similar symptoms, that does not resolve with bedrest, and that is severe enough to reduce or impair average daily activity below fifty percent of the patient's premorbid activity level for a period of at least six months." (2) Exclusion of other plausible disorders "by thorough evaluation, based on history, physical examination, and appropriate laboratory findings."

The CDC's symptom criteria include onset of the symptom complex over a few hours or days and ten other symptoms. (These are listed first under What Are the Symptoms?) The CDC's physical criteria, which must be documented on at least two occasions, at least one month apart, are low-grade fever, nonexudative pharyngitis (sore throat), and palpable or tender lymph nodes. The CDC has stated that this definition is only "an operational concept" and it may therefore fail to include many persons who have this syndrome.

Although the CDC case definition is in some sense "official" (and legitimizes the illness), it is considered provisional because it is based on symptoms which can be produced by other diseases and on the exclusion of such diseases. Fortunately, pioneering CFIDS clinicians and researchers are making great strides in identifying specific objective markers for diagnosing CFIDS and for assessing patient treatment response. As reported in the *CFIDS Chronicle* (see especially "CFIDS: The Diagnosis of a Distinct Illness," September 1992), physicians and scientists in Australia, California, Canada, Florida, North Carolina, Texas, Wisconsin, and elsewhere are developing an array of tests which are increasingly sensitive and specific for CFIDS. As the cause and mechanism of this disease become clear, so will the clinical and laboratory parameters which define CFIDS. Ultimately, conclusive diagnostic standards will be developed and accepted.

Unfortunately, many physicians are not very familiar with CFIDS and have difficulty diagnosing it. Others still do not even know that the illness exists. As a result, PWCs are often misdiagnosed, sometimes as having psychosomatic or affective disorder because such conditions are also diagnosed by exclusion in many cases.

What Are the Symptoms? PWCs experience symptoms which tend to be *individualistic* and to fluctuate in severity. They may include profound or prolonged fatigue, especially after exercise levels that would have been easily tolerated before; low-grade fever; sore throat; painful lymph nodes; muscle weakness; muscle discomfort or myalgia (pain or aching); sleep disturbance (hypersomnia or insomnia); headaches of a new type, severity, or pattern; migratory arthralgia without joint swelling or redness; neuropsychologic problems, including photophobia, transient visual scotomata (spots), forgetfulness, irritability, confusion, difficulty thinking, inability to concentrate, and depression; other cognitive function problems (such as spatial disorientation and dyslogia—impairment of speech and/or reasoning), visual disturbances (blurring, sensitivity to light, eye pain, frequent prescription changes), and psychological problems (anxiety, panic attacks, personality changes, emotional lability); chills and night sweats; shortness of breath; dizziness and balance problems; sensitivity to heat and cold; intolerance of alcohol; irregular heartbeat; abdominal pain, diarrhea, irritable bowel; low temperature; numbness of or burning in the face or extremities; dryness of the mouth and eyes (sicca syndrome); hearing disorders or sensitivity; menstrual problems including PMS and endometriosis; hypersensitivity of the skin; chest pains; rashes; allergies and sensitivities to odors, chemicals, and medications; weight changes without changes in diet; hair loss; lightheadedness—feeling "in a fog"; fainting; muscle twitching; and seizures.

How Can CFIDS Be Treated? What Is the Prognosis? No primary therapy has been proven to cure CFIDS. However, trials are underway with Ampligen, Kutapressin, and other experimental treatment methods. In addition, some symptoms frequently can be alleviated by prescription drugs (such as Klonopin, Prozac, Sinequan, Xanax, and Zantac), but these must be carefully tailored to the needs of each individual and often must be taken in unusually low dosages. Also, avoidance of environmental irritants and certain foods can sometimes relieve symptoms and many PWCs claim to have benefited from nutritional therapies. A significant percentage of PWCs show marked improvement over time. But many remain ill or cycle through a continuing series of remissions and relapses. The symptoms in severely affected PWCs can be devastating and result in prolonged interruption of work and family life. Some researchers believe that PWCs may also be at greater risk of developing other illnesses. However, the extent to which CFIDS may be progressive or degenerative is not yet known. For additional information on treatment options and prognosis, see the *CFIDS Chronicle* or call the CFIDS Information Line.

Is CFIDS Contagious? It is probable that the viruses and/or other agents that trigger CFIDS are easily transmitted. CFIDS has been reported in many children and monogamous adults and "clustering" of cases in families, workplaces, and communities also seems to occur. Anecdotal reports exist of pets of CFIDS patients getting unusual diseases. However, whether a person develops CFIDS is believed to be a function of how his/her system deals with the causative agent(s). Most people in close contact with CFIDS patients have not developed the illness.

How Does One Live with CFIDS? Persons with CFIDS must identify their limits and learn to operate within them. Symptoms tend to be aggravated by physical or emotional stress, and improved by rest. Those who accept the fact that they have a chronic illness and turn down the rheostat on their lives generally cope better than those who deny reality. Many PWCs overcome the sense of isolation and helplessness common to the disease by joining support groups and working to help each other. In telephone calls, newsletters, journals, and at meetings and conferences, they share experiences, exchange information, and learn from each other. PWCs often find an equilibrium point at which they can function. *As in combating any chronic illness, a positive, hopeful attitude is essential.*

Which Physicians Understand CFIDS? Finding a physician knowledgeable about CFIDS can be difficult. The symptoms are not organ-specific, and no single medical discipline has embraced the disease. Individuals who have been diagnosed with CFIDS are excellent sources of referrals and a Physicians Honor Roll of CFIDS clinicians (nominated by their patients) is available from the CFIDS Association of America. In addition, a list of physicians knowledgeable about CFIDS is maintained by most local support groups. However, if you already have a good relationship with a doctor, you should urge him/her to develop an understanding of this disease.

For more information, write to the CFIDS Association of America, Inc., PO Box 220398, Charlotte, NC 28222-0398, or call 800-442-3437 (fax 704-365-9755). The number of the CFIDS Information Line is 900-896-2343.

CURRENT LITERATURE ON CFS/ON-LINE SUPPORT SERVICES

ARTICLES AND BOOKS

Bell, David S., M.D. *The Doctor's Guide to Chronic Fatigue Syndrome.* Reading, MA: Addison-Wesley, 1994. Dr. Bell, regarded as one of the world's leading CFIDS experts, provides a definitive guide to the history, symptoms, effects, theories, treatment, and ongoing research of this devastating illness.

Berne, Katrina H., Ph.D. *Running on Empty.* Alameda, CA: Hunter House, 1992. Dr. Berne draws on her experience as a PWC, CFIDS therapist, and speaker in writing this well-researched thesis on what little is known about CFIDS. She addresses nearly every aspect of recognizing and living with CFIDS.

Collinge, William, Ph.D. *Recovering from Chronic Fatigue Syndrome: A Guide to Self-Empowerment.* New York: Putnam, 1993. Dr. Collinge, creator of the first mind/body program for CFIDS, details his approach to healing.

Cowley, Jeffrey. "Chronic Fatigue Syndrome: A Modern Medical Mystery." *Newsweek,* November 12, 1990. Seven pages of *Newsweek*'s cover story are devoted to an in-depth study of the disease, including patient profiles and the latest research.

Feiden, Karyn. *Hope and Help for Chronic Fatigue Syndrome.* Englewood Cliffs, NJ: Prentice Hall, 1992. This book provides great insight into the experience of having CFIDS and the key strategies for regaining control over your life.

Johnston, Hillary. "Journey into Fear—The Growing Nightmare of Epstein-Barr Virus." *Rolling Stone,* July 30/August 13, 1987. These highly personal stories chronicle the effort of a journalist stricken by CFIDS to comprehend both the disease and the breadth of the epidemic. They include interviews with several prominent CFIDS researchers.

Shepherd, Charles, Dr. *Living with ME.* London: Cedar, 1992. Dr. Shepherd describes ME (myalgic encephalomyelitis—the British term for chronic fatigue syndrome), discusses practical methods for coping, and comments on various treatments.

ON-LINE SUPPORT SERVICES

The following commercial on-line services all provide access to the Internet:

Prodigy (800-776-3449) has a very active CFS discussion and support group, with hundreds of notes posted daily.

GEnie (800-638-9636) has a category devoted to CFS, a library of files, and a monthly conference.

America Online (800-827-6364) has a live chat session every week on CFS and a library of files, and notes about CFS are posted in the Disabilities area.

CompuServe (800-848-8199) has a CFS discussion in the Health and Fitness forum and a library of files.

Internet has the following resources:

CFS-L is a discussion group consisting of people with CFS from all over the world. For information on joining, contact the moderator at CFS-L-REQUEST@LIST.NIH.GOV.

CFS-News is an electronic newsletter providing the latest news on CFS. To subscribe, send a message to CFS-NEWS@LIST.NIH.GOV.

Catharsis is an electronic newsmagazine that focuses on health, intellect, and creativity. To subscribe, contact the editor at CATHAR-M@SJUVM.STJOHNS.EDU.

CFS Newswire is a service that provides patients, support group leaders, and newsletter editors with a way to exchange news articles. Contact the CFS/ME Computer Networking Project at CFS-ME@SJUVM.STJOHNS.EDU.

Other Resources: There are local electronic bulletin board systems (BBS) that may be free or have a nominal fee. For a listing of these BBS and other information about electronic resources, contact the CFS/ME Computer Networking Project at CFS-ME@SJUVM.STJOHNS.EDU, or send a stamped, self-addressed envelope to PO Box 2397, Washington, DC 20013.

INDEX

TK stands for Tim Kenny.